Balanced Living

5-Minute Daily Mindful Routines for Seniors

Scott Anthony

WISEGUY
MEDIA

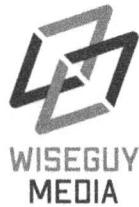

For more information, contact : Wiseguy Media

http://www.wiseguymediapublication.com

Cover design by Valentina Ikiana

Library of Congress Active Collection

ISBN - Paperback: **979-8-9892846-3-4**

First Edition: November 2023

Contents

About the Author

Scott is a dedicated advocate for health and wellness. With a genuine passion for promoting well-being, he has authored several books that reflect his commitment to helping individuals lead healthier lives. Scott's journey into the world of holistic health has been multifaceted, as he has not only penned insightful works but also hosted talk shows alongside naturopathic doctors, offering a holistic approach to health and wellness. Through these collaborative endeavors, he has had the privilege of engaging with experts in the field and sharing their wisdom with a wider audience. Scott's dedication to the holistic principles of well-being shines through in his work, and his desire to empower individuals to take charge of their health is both evident and inspiring. This book is a testament to his unwavering commitment to the cause of holistic wellness, and it is an invitation for you to join him on this enlightening journey.

Introduction

Let's face it, as we get older, we tend to slow down. Friends move, interests change, and we find a new routine in front of a TV to keep is entertained. But all the research shows that when we slow down and isolate see a reduction in health, energy and longevity. Taking on big exercise routines or other activities might seem daunting. But the key to wellness is about small steps that keep us well balanced in all areas of our lives.

If you've been on the lookout for ways to feel better, boost your mood, and stay sharp, you're in the right place. We've ditched the complicated jargon and rigid routines; this book is about making life easier, one small step at a time.

Picture this: a day where you feel steady on your feet, calm in your mind, and ready to tackle anything life throws your way. That's the magic of balance, and here we will show you how just five minutes a day can get you there.

But wait, what's the big deal about balance anyway? Well, it's not just about not wobbling when you stand up (though that's important too!). Balance means feeling in control, steady, and centered, physically, mentally, and emotionally. It's the secret sauce for a life well-lived, especially for us seasoned folks.

Now, we're not here to throw complicated fitness routines your way or bore you with heaps of science. Nope, this is all about simplicity, fun, and brightening each day. We've turned balance exercises into easy-peasy daily routines. You can do them while brewing your morning coffee or waiting for your favorite TV show to start; no sweat, right?

And we've sprinkled in a dash of mindfulness because, trust us, it's like a superpower. Mindfulness is all about being present, feeling calm, and letting go of stress. We've got your back with soothing illustrations to make it even more enjoyable.

So, if you're ready to feel better than ever, join us on this journey to balanced living. Say goodbye to stress and hello to a happier, healthier you!

Chapter 1:

The Power of Balance Routines

Welcome to the world of daily balance routines, a simple yet powerful concept that can transform your life. In this introduction, we'll break down what balance routines are, why they matter, and how they can enhance your daily routine. Don't worry; we're going to keep things simple and easy to understand, perfect for seniors like us who want to add a little more balance to our lives.

Imagine your life as a delicate dance between different aspects: your physical well-being, mental clarity, emotional stability, and social connections. Just like a symphony, all these elements need to be in harmony to create beautiful music. Balance routines are the choreography that keeps this dance graceful and fulfilling, especially as we navigate the journey of aging.

What are balance routines?

Balance routines are small, intentional practices or habits that you incorporate into your daily life to promote equilibrium and well-being. They're not rigid rules or complicated routines; instead, they're like gentle nudges that guide you toward a more balanced and contented existence.

You might be wondering, "What exactly are balance routines?" Well, think of them as little routines or practices that help us find harmony in our daily lives. They're like our secret weapons for feeling better physically, mentally, and emotionally.

Why are balance routines so important?

Let me break it down for you. Balance routines help you:

- ★ **Stay Energized:** Balancing our energy levels is crucial as we age. These routines can help us stay active and vibrant, so we have the energy to do the things we love.

★ **Reduce Stress:** Life can get pretty hectic, right? Balance routines can be your go-to stress busters. They'll help you relax and find peace in the midst of chaos.

★ **Boost Health:** Maintaining good health is a top priority. By incorporating balance routines into your routine, you can support your physical and mental well-being.

★ **Stay Connected:** Balance routines can also be a way to connect with friends and family. Sharing these practices with loved ones can bring you closer together.

Now, here's the fun part. There's no one-size-fits-all when it comes to balancing routines. You get to choose what works best for you. It could be something as simple as a morning walk, practicing deep breathing, or even sipping a cup of herbal tea in the evening.

We will explore different balance routines and how you can easily incorporate them into your daily life. No need to worry about complicated instructions or strict schedules. We're keeping things relaxed and flexible.

Remember, the power of balance routines lies in consistency. By making them a part of your routine, you can experience a more balanced, happier, and healthier life. So, get ready to discover the magic of balance routines, and let's embark on this journey together.

Now, we will go into routines in more depth in a bit but for now let's dive into some simple and enjoyable and mindful balance routines that you can start incorporating into your life today:

★ **Morning Stretch:** Start your day with a gentle morning stretch. It's a great way to wake up your body and get your blood flowing. You don't need to be a yoga expert; just reach for the sky, touch your toes, and twist your torso gently. This can help ease any stiffness and set a positive tone for the day.

★ **Daily Gratitude:** Take a moment each morning to reflect on the things you're grateful for. It could be as simple as the warm sunlight streaming through your window or the taste of your morning coffee. Practicing gratitude can boost your mood and help you stay positive.

★ **Nature Connection:** Spend some time in nature, even if it's just in your backyard or at a nearby park. Take a leisurely stroll, listen to the birds, or watch the leaves rustle in the wind. Nature has a calming effect that can help you find balance and inner peace.

★ **Mindful Breathing:** Whenever you're feeling stressed or anxious, practice some mindful breathing. Close your eyes, take a deep breath through your nose, and exhale slowly through your mouth. Repeat this a few times, focusing on your breath. It's a simple way to regain composure and reduce stress.

★ **Tea Time:** Make tea drinking a daily routine. Choose herbal teas like chamomile or peppermint, which have calming properties. Sipping on a warm cup of tea can be incredibly soothing and comforting.

★ **Evening Reflection:** Before bed, take a few minutes to reflect on your day. Think about your accomplishments and the positive moments. This can help you go to sleep with a sense of contentment and peace.

★ **Stay Social:** Balance routines can also involve spending quality time with loved ones. Whether it's a phone call, a visit, or a simple game night with friends or family, maintaining social connections is vital for emotional well-being.

★ **Good Night's Sleep:** Establish a bedtime routine that helps you unwind and get a good night's sleep. Turn off the TV and dim the lights an hour before bedtime. Read a book or practice some gentle stretches to relax your body.

★ **Community Involvement:** Volunteering or participating in community events can bring a sense of purpose and fulfillment. It's also a great way to meet new people and strengthen your social connections.

These balance routines are like building blocks, helping you create a well-rounded and fulfilling life. Remember, there is no need to rush or feel pressured to do them all at once. Start with one or two that resonate with you, and gradually add more as you feel comfortable. The key is to make them a part of your daily routine, so they become second nature. Over time, you will likely notice positive changes in your physical and mental well-being.

Balance is all about finding what works best for you and your unique journey. It is about embracing the simple joys in life and taking care of yourself in a way that brings harmony to your days. So, go ahead and experiment with these routines, and let us continue this path to a balanced and happy life together!

So, there you have it, a few easy-to-follow balance routines to get you started on your journey to a more harmonious and balanced life. This is just the beginning, and there is so much more to explore. Stay tuned for more simple and senior-friendly tips in the chapters to come.

The Significance of Balance in Seniors' Lives

Balance is a cornerstone of a fulfilling and healthy life, and it holds particular significance in the lives of seniors. As we age, the importance of balance becomes even more pronounced, influencing various aspects of well-being. Let's explore why balance is so significant for seniors:

Physical Well-Being: Maintaining physical balance is crucial for seniors. A steady and balanced body helps prevent falls and injuries, which can have severe consequences as we age. Balance exercises and activities can improve muscle strength, coordination, and stability, enabling seniors to stay active and independent.

Fall Prevention: Falls are a leading cause of injuries among seniors, often resulting in fractures and hospitalizations. Balance training and exercises can reduce the risk of falls by enhancing posture, equilibrium, and reaction time, providing seniors with greater confidence in their day-to-day activities.

Pain Management: Balance can play a role in managing chronic pain conditions, such as arthritis. Proper alignment and balance can reduce stress on joints, leading to less pain and discomfort.

Mental Clarity: Physical balance is intertwined with mental clarity. When we feel physically stable, our minds are clearer, allowing seniors to stay engaged, make sound decisions, and enjoy a better overall quality of life.

Emotional Well-Being: Balance extends beyond the physical realm; it also affects emotional stability. Seniors who maintain balance in their lives often report lower levels of stress, anxiety, and depression. Balance routines can be a source of comfort, helping seniors find solace and peace in their daily routines.

Social Connection: Seniors who maintain a balanced lifestyle are more likely to engage in social activities and maintain strong relationships with friends and family. Balance routines, such as group exercises or regular outings, provide opportunities for socialization, reducing feelings of isolation and loneliness.

Longevity: Leading a balanced life can contribute to a longer and more fulfilling lifespan. Seniors who prioritize balance tend to enjoy better overall health, fewer health complications, and a greater sense of purpose.

Sense of Independence: Perhaps one of the most significant aspects for seniors, balance contributes to independence. By maintaining physical and emotional balance, seniors can continue to live life on their terms, staying self-reliant and active in their communities.

Adaptability: As we age, our bodies and circumstances change. Balance routines help seniors adapt to these changes with greater ease. They provide a framework for adjusting to new routines, medical conditions, or living situations, allowing seniors to maintain a sense of equilibrium in the face of life's transitions.

Sense of Achievement: Setting and achieving balance-related goals, no matter how small, can boost self-esteem and a sense of accomplishment. Seniors can take pride in their ability to incorporate balanced routines into their daily lives, fostering a positive outlook and motivation to continue their journey.

Spiritual Fulfillment: For many seniors, balance routines extend beyond the physical and mental realms to encompass spiritual well-being. Engaging in practices like meditation, prayer, or spending time in nature can provide a sense of inner peace and purpose, nurturing the soul.

Resilience: Seniors who maintain balance are often better equipped to face life's challenges and setbacks. They develop resilience, and the ability to bounce back from adversity, which can be especially important in later life when dealing with health issues or the loss of loved ones.

Legacy and Wisdom: By prioritizing balance in their lives, seniors can serve as role models and mentors to younger generations, passing down their wisdom and knowledge. This legacy can be a source of pride and fulfillment, reinforcing their sense of purpose.

The significance of balance in seniors' lives cannot be overstated. It influences their physical health, emotional well-being, social connections, and overall quality of life. Balance routines and practices provide seniors with the tools to age gracefully, stay active and independent, and find fulfillment in their later years. It's an ongoing journey, and the benefits are well worth the effort, contributing to a vibrant and rewarding senior life. Balance is not just a physical concept; it encompasses all aspects of seniors' lives. It directly impacts their physical health, emotional well-being, and social connections. Seniors who prioritize balance through daily routines and activities can lead more fulfilling, active, and independent lives. It's a vital component of aging gracefully and maintaining a high quality of life throughout the senior years.

Benefits of Incorporating Mindfulness into Daily Routines

Let's talk about the benefits of adding a little mindfulness into your daily life. So, what is mindfulness anyway? Well, it's like giving your mind a little vacation from all the hustle and bustle of daily life. It's about paying attention to the present moment and being fully aware of what's happening around you. Here are some of the great things it can do for you:

Reducing Stress: Mindfulness can help you relax and lower stress levels. When you take a moment to breathe and focus on the now, it's like hitting the reset button for your mind.

Improved Focus: Do you ever find your mind wandering when you're trying to concentrate on something? Mindfulness can sharpen your focus and make it easier to get things done.

Happier Thoughts: When you're mindful, you're more likely to have positive thoughts and a brighter outlook on life. It's like giving your brain a dose of happiness.

Better Relationships: Mindfulness can also improve your relationships with others. When you're fully present in conversations, people appreciate it, and it can strengthen your connections.

Pain Management: Some people find that mindfulness helps them manage physical pain better. It's not a magic cure, but it can make it more bearable.

What activities would be considered Mindful

Remember that mindfulness is about being in the moment. Slowing time down to really focus the present, it's the only thing we have control over. Some of these mindful activities get us going in the right direction.

Morning Mindfulness: Start your day on the right foot. Instead of rushing out of bed, take a moment to focus on your breathing. As you inhale and exhale, think about how your body feels. This simple practice can set a calm tone for the day ahead.

Mindful Meals: Eating can be a great time to practice mindfulness. When you sit down to eat, pay attention to the flavors, textures, and smells of your food. Slow down, savor each bite, and enjoy your meal more fully.

Nature Connection: If you can, spend some time in nature. Whether it's a park, a garden, or simply your backyard, being in natural surroundings can be incredibly calming. Listen to the birds, feel the breeze, and soak up the beauty around you.

Breathing Breaks: Throughout the day, take short breaks to focus on your breath. It's as easy as taking three deep breaths and clearing your mind for a minute or two. This can help reduce stress and re-energize you.

Mindful Walking: When you're out for a walk, whether it's a leisurely stroll or just going from one place to another, pay attention to your steps. Feel the ground beneath your feet and the movement of your body. It's like a moving meditation.

Gratitude Journal: Before bed, jot down a few things you're grateful for that happened during the day. It could be as simple as a delicious meal, a smile from a friend, or a beautiful sunset. Reflecting on these moments can boost your mood.

Guided Meditation: If you're new to mindfulness, there are plenty of easy-to-follow guided meditation apps or videos available online. They'll walk you through the process, making it a breeze to get started.

So, how can you start incorporating mindfulness into your daily routine? It's as easy as taking a few minutes each day to sit quietly, breathe deeply, and focus on what's happening right now. You don't need any special equipment or training; just a willingness to give it a try.

Remember, mindfulness is all about taking things one step at a time and being kind to yourself. It's not about being perfect; it's about being present. So, go ahead and give it a shot. Your mind and body will thank you for it! there's no rush, and there's no wrong way to do mindfulness. The key is to find what works best for you and make it a regular part of your routine.

Setting the Stage for a Holistic Approach to Well-Being

Let's talk about something super important: taking care of ourselves in a way that makes us feel good all around. We call it a "holistic approach to well-being," but don't let the big words scare you; it's just about looking after your body and mind in a way that covers all the bases.

Picture this: you're like a puzzle, and each piece of the puzzle represents a different aspect of your well-being. There's the physical piece, the mental piece, the emotional piece, and even the social piece. So, let's break it down:

- **Physical Well-Being:** This is all about keeping your body in good shape. It means eating nutritious foods, getting some exercise (even a simple walk counts!), and getting enough sleep. Think of it as fueling and resting your body so it can do its job.

- **Mental Well-Being:** Your mind needs love too! Take breaks, do things you enjoy, and try relaxation techniques like deep breathing or simple meditation. It's like giving your brain a spa day.

- **Emotional Well-Being:** Emotions are totally normal, but it's important to deal with them in a healthy way. Talk to friends or family if you need to, or even a professional. Don't bottle it up – it's like letting out steam from a kettle.

- **Social Well-Being:** We're social creatures and being with others can lift our spirits. Spend time with friends, join clubs or groups, and stay connected. It's like adding a little sprinkle of joy to your life.

- **Nutrition**: Eating well doesn't have to be complicated. Think of it as adding colors to your plate – lots of veggies, fruits, whole grains, and lean proteins. But don't forget to enjoy your favorite treats in moderation because a little indulgence can be good for the soul.

- **Exercise:** If the idea of hitting the gym sounds daunting, don't worry! You can keep it simple with activities like dancing, gardening, or even stretching at home. The key is to find something you enjoy, so you'll stick with it. Remember, staying active is like giving your body a little love tap.

- **Positive Thinking:** Try to catch those negative thoughts and replace them with more positive ones. It's like giving your mind a sunny day to bask in. Surround yourself with positive people, too – they can lift you up when you need it most.

- **Balance:** Life can get hectic, but it's essential to find a balance that works for you. Prioritize your well-being without overloading your schedule. It's like juggling, but you don't want to drop any of your happiness balls.

- **Laugh and Have Fun:** Laughter truly is the best medicine. Watch a funny movie, spend time with loved ones, or pick up a hobby that brings you joy. Having fun is like adding a little sparkle to your day.

- **Learn and Grow:** Keep your mind active by learning new things or pursuing your interests. It could be reading, taking up a new hobby, or even going back to school. Learning is like watering your brain; it helps it thrive.

Remember, you don't have to tackle all these aspects at once. Small steps can lead to big changes in your well-being. So, take it easy, be kind to yourself, and enjoy the journey to a happier and healthier you. Your well-being is worth every effort, and you've got a whole world of support and resources to help you along the way!

Scott Anthony

Chapter 2

Building your Daily Routine

How to Create a Personalized Daily Routine

Start Small: Begin by choosing just one or two simple activities you'd like to incorporate into your daily routine. These could be activities that you genuinely enjoy or ones that bring a sense of calm and well-being. Examples include enjoying a cup of herbal tea, doing a crossword puzzle, or taking a short stroll around your garden.

Set a Time: It's important to establish a specific time for your daily routine. This helps create a routine. For instance, you might decide to have your quiet time with a cup of tea right after breakfast, or you could reserve a few minutes before bedtime to read a book.

Make it Meaningful: Your daily routine should hold personal meaning for you. It could be something that helps you relax, reflect, or simply start your day on a positive note. For example, practicing deep breathing exercises, spending a few moments in quiet reflection, or even tending to a small indoor plant can all be meaningful activities.

Stay Consistent: Consistency is the key to turning your daily routine into a habit. Try your best to stick to your chosen time and activity each day. Over time, it will become second nature.

No Pressure: Don't put too much pressure on yourself. If you happen to miss a day due to unforeseen circumstances or simply not feeling up to it, that's completely okay. Just pick it up again the next day. Your routine should be a source of joy, not stress.

Adapt and Evolve: As you go along, you might find that your interests or needs change. Feel free to adjust your daily routine accordingly. It's a flexible concept that can evolve with you. If you discover new activities that bring you happiness or relaxation, incorporate them.

Reflect and Appreciate: Take a moment to reflect on the benefits of your daily routine. How does it make you feel? What positive changes have you noticed in your life? Express gratitude for the simple pleasures it brings and the sense of routine it provides.

Share or Invite Others: If you find that your daily routine brings you joy, consider sharing it with a friend or inviting a loved one to join you. Sharing these moments can strengthen connections and create special memories together.

Be Patient and Gentle: Understand that building a daily routine takes time and patience. It may take a few weeks or even months for it to become a seamless part of your routine. Be gentle with yourself during this process and celebrate small victories along the way.

Record Your Progress: Optionally, you can keep a journal to record your daily routine experiences. Note how you feel before and after, any insights you gain, or any adjustments you make. It can be a wonderful way to track your journey and see how far you've come.

Seek Inspiration: If you ever feel like you need fresh ideas or motivation, don't hesitate to seek inspiration from books, articles, or friends who also have their daily routines. Sometimes, a new perspective can rejuvenate your practice.

Stay Open to Change: Life is dynamic, and your needs and preferences may evolve over time. Don't be afraid to adapt your routine accordingly. What brings you comfort and joy today might be different from what you need tomorrow.

Enjoy the Process: Lastly, always keep in mind that the purpose of your daily routine is to make your day more enjoyable and intentional. It's not a chore; it's a gift to yourself. So, approach it with a sense of enjoyment and anticipation. Look forward to this special time you've set aside for yourself each day.

In summary, creating a personalized daily routine is a beautiful way to add structure and positivity to your life, without it feeling like a daunting task. It's about taking simple steps to make your days more intentional and enjoyable. Keep it meaningful, stay consistent, and remember that it's a journey meant to enhance your well-being. Embrace it with enthusiasm, and let it bring a sense of fulfillment to your daily life. The key is to find activities that resonate with you and make your days a bit brighter and more intentional. Have fun with it, and cherish these moments you've set aside for yourself.

Choosing the Right Time and Space

When it comes to choosing the right time and space for various activities, it's all about finding what works best for you. Whether you're planning your day, organizing an event, or just trying to relax, here are some simple tips to consider, especially if you're a senior:

When it comes to choosing the right time and space for various activities, it's all about finding what works best for you. Whether you're planning your day, organizing an event, or just trying to relax, here are some simple tips to consider, especially if you're a senior:

Consider Your Energy Levels: Thinking about your energy levels is an essential part of choosing the right time and space for your activities, especially as a senior. Here are some simple tips to help you make the most of your energy. Many seniors find that their energy levels are highest in the morning. This is a great time to tackle tasks that require focus and concentration, like paying bills, reading, or doing puzzles.

Afternoons can sometimes be a bit of a slump for energy. Consider taking a short nap if you're feeling tired. It can do wonders to recharge your batteries for the rest of the day. In the evenings, opt for more relaxed activities. This is a good time to watch your favorite TV shows, chat with friends and family, or enjoy a soothing cup of tea.

Dehydration can make you feel tired, so be sure to drink enough water throughout the day to keep your energy levels up. Snack on healthy foods like fruits, nuts, or yogurt to keep your energy stable between meals. Gentle exercises like stretching or a short walk can boost your energy without exhausting you. Don't overexert yourself. If you have a busy day planned, make sure to schedule breaks to rest and recharge.

Your body will tell you when it's time for rest or activity. Pay attention to how you feel and adjust your plans accordingly. By considering your energy levels and planning your activities accordingly, you can make the most of your day while avoiding unnecessary fatigue. Remember, it's all about finding the right balance for you.

Avoid Rush Hours: Avoiding rush hours is a smart choice, especially if you want to make your outings more relaxed and less stressful, especially as a senior. Here's why and how to do it. Rush hours are often characterized by heavy traffic and crowded spaces. By avoiding these times, you can reduce stress and anxiety associated with navigating busy roads or crowded public transport. As a senior, it's important to prioritize your safety. Rush hours can be chaotic, increasing the risk of accidents. Choosing quieter times can help keep you safe.

Rush hours can result in wasted time spent stuck in traffic or waiting in long lines. By avoiding these periods, you can save valuable time for other activities. If you know you need to go out, plan your trips during non-peak hours. Consider going out earlier in the morning or later in the afternoon when traffic tends to be lighter. Apps like Google Maps or Waze can provide real-time traffic updates. Use them to find the best times to travel and alternate routes if necessary.

If possible, see if you can work from home or schedule appointments during off-peak hours to avoid commuting during rush times. Grocery shopping and other errands can be more pleasant when stores are less crowded. Try going during weekday mornings or mid-week when it's quieter.

If you rely on public transportation, check the schedule for less crowded times. Mid-morning or mid-afternoon can be quieter than the morning and evening rush. Don't hesitate to ask a friend or family member to accompany you on outings, especially during busier times. They can help with navigation and carrying items. Keep an eye on local news or traffic reports to stay informed about road closures or special events that may impact traffic.

Avoiding rush hours isn't just about convenience; it can also contribute to a safer and more enjoyable experience when you're out and about. So, take a little extra time to plan your activities, and you'll likely find that your outings are much more pleasant.

Comfortable Spaces: "Weather Matters" and "Comfortable Spaces" are two crucial aspects to consider when you're planning your day, especially as a senior. Let's break down these ideas: Check the weather forecast before heading out. Dress in layers during unpredictable weather, and don't forget your umbrella or sun hat when needed.

Extreme weather conditions like heavy rain, snow, or extreme heat can be risky for seniors. Consider postponing outdoor activities during severe weather to ensure your safety. On pleasant days, take advantage of the good weather. Go for a walk, have a picnic, or do some gardening to soak up the sunshine and fresh air. Keep an eye on weather updates, especially if you have any outdoor plans. Sudden changes in weather can affect your day, so it's best to be prepared.

Comfortable Spaces: Make sure your living space is organized and clutter-free. This can prevent accidents and make daily activities more comfortable. Invest in ergonomic furniture and accessories if needed. Chairs with good back support and adjustable tables can help you stay comfortable while reading, using the computer. Install handrails or grab bars in the bathroom and along staircases for added safety. Non-slip mats can prevent slips and falls.

Create a cozy corner in your home where you can relax with a good book, enjoy a cup of tea, or simply unwind. Comfortable seating and good lighting are essential. Ensure your home is at a comfortable temperature. Use heating or cooling systems as needed and consider using fans or blankets to stay comfortable. Surround yourself with items that bring you joy and comfort, whether it's family photos, favorite artwork, or soothing colors.

Remember, there's no one-size-fits-all answer when it comes to choosing the right time and space. It's about finding what suits you best and making your everyday life as enjoyable and comfortable as possible. Don't hesitate to ask for help or advice from friends, family, or caregivers if you're uncertain about any decisions.

Remember, the weather and your living space can significantly impact your well-being and daily activities. By paying attention to both of these factors, you can enhance your comfort, safety, and overall quality of life.

Establishing Achievable Goals and Intentions

Setting goals and intentions is a fundamental part of leading a fulfilling life. Whether you're a senior looking to stay active and engaged, or you're simply seeking to make positive changes, having clear goals can help you stay motivated and focused. In this guide, we'll explore the importance of setting achievable goals and intentions and provide simple, practical tips to help you get started. Remember, it's never too late to dream, plan, and achieve your aspirations!

Setting goals and intentions can bring numerous benefits to your life, no matter your age. Here's why it's essential: Having clear goals provides a sense of purpose and direction. It gives you something to work toward and wakes you up with a reason to start your day. When you have a goal, it's easier to stay motivated. Goals can serve as a source of inspiration, keeping you moving forward even when obstacles arise.

Goals help you concentrate your efforts on specific tasks and priorities. This can lead to increased productivity and a greater sense of accomplishment. Achieving your goals boosts your self-esteem and confidence. It reminds you that you're capable of making positive changes in your life. Setting and achieving goals can lead to personal growth and development. It encourages you to step out of your comfort zone and learn new things.

Before we dive into the process of setting goals, let's explore the various types of goals and intentions you can consider: Short-term goals are those you can accomplish in the near future, often within a few days or weeks. Long-term goals, on the other hand, may take months or even years to achieve. A good balance of both types can help you stay motivated.

Personal goals are related to your individual desires and aspirations. They might include improving your health, learning a new skill, or traveling to a specific destination.

Social goals involve your interactions with others. These could include building better relationships with family and friends or becoming more active in your community.

Financial goals relate to your financial well-being. This might involve saving for retirement, paying off debts, or budgeting more effectively. Health and wellness goals are focused on improving your physical and mental well-being. They can include exercise, a balanced diet, stress management, and regular check-ups.

These goals center around your hobbies and interests, such as taking up a new hobby, mastering a craft, or exploring a new passion. Now that you understand the importance of setting goals and the different types you can consider, let's explore how to set achievable goals. Remember, the key is to keep it simple and realistic. Make your goals as specific as possible. Instead of saying, "I want to get in shape," try, "I want to walk for 30 minutes every day."

You should be able to measure your progress. This allows you to track your achievements and stay motivated. For instance, if your goal is to read more, set a target of finishing a certain number of books per month. Give yourself a timeframe to work within. Having a deadline adds urgency and helps you stay focused. For example, "I will declutter my garage by the end of the month."

Set goals that are attainable given your current circumstances and resources. If you haven't run in years, don't aim to complete a marathon in a month. Start with a goal like running a mile without stopping. Putting your goals in writing makes them feel more concrete. You can create a list or a vision board to help visualize your aspirations.

While setting goals is important, it's equally crucial to establish intentions. Intentions are the mindset and attitude you bring to your daily life. Here's why they matter: Intentions guide your daily actions and decisions. They serve as a compass, helping you stay aligned with your values and goals.

Setting positive intentions can lead to a more optimistic outlook on life. For instance, if you intend to approach challenges with resilience, you'll be better equipped to handle setbacks. Intentions encourage mindfulness, the practice of being fully present in the moment. This can reduce stress and enhance your overall well-being.

Intentions can improve your relationships with others. If you set an intention to be more patient, you're likely to communicate more effectively and empathetically. Now that you understand the importance of both goals and intentions, it's time to put everything into practice. Here's a step-by-step guide:

Start by thinking about your core values and what matters most to you. Your goals and intentions should align with these values. What areas of your life do you want to improve? Is it your health, relationships, or personal growth? Make a list of your top priorities. Based on your priorities, set specific, measurable, and achievable goals. Write them down and include deadlines.

Establish positive intentions that will guide your actions as you work toward your goals. For example, if your goal is to improve your health, your intention could be to prioritize self-care and make healthy choices. Break your goals into smaller, actionable steps. This makes them more manageable and less intimidating. Share your goals and intentions with a trusted friend or family member who can help keep you accountable. You can also track your progress in a journal or on a calendar. Don't forget to celebrate your successes, no matter how small. Rewarding yourself reinforces positive behavior.

Setting achievable goals and intentions can have a profound impact on your life as a senior. It gives you a sense of purpose, motivation, and direction. Whether you want to improve your health, build stronger relationships, or pursue your passions, the key is to start small, stay focused, and never stop dreaming. Remember, it's never too late to live a life filled with purpose and meaning.

Integrating Balance Exercises into Daily Life

Sure, let's talk about adding some balance exercises to your daily routine. It's not too complicated, and it can really help improve your stability and prevent falls.

Stand on One Leg: Start with something simple. Find a sturdy chair or countertop to hold onto, and then lift one leg off the ground. Try to balance on the other leg for 10-15 seconds, then switch to the other leg. As you get more comfortable, you can try to let go of the support for short periods.

Heel-to-Toe Walk: Imagine you're walking on a tightrope. Take a step forward by placing the heel of one foot directly in front of the toes of the other foot. Keep going, heel to toe, for about 20 steps. If you need to, you can have a wall or a friend nearby for support.

Mini Leg Raises: While bracing yourself and standing, lift one leg a few inches off the ground and hold it for a few seconds. Lower it down and switch to the other leg. Do this 10 times on each leg. It's like a mini leg workout!

Sit to Stand: This one's great for your legs and balance. Sit down on a sturdy chair, then stand up without using your hands or arms for support. Sit back down and repeat 10 times. As you get stronger, try doing it without sitting all the way down.

Tai Chi or Yoga: These are gentle exercises that promote balance, flexibility, and relaxation. You can find beginner classes online or in your community. They're a great way to stay active and improve your balance.

Practice Regularly: The key to improving your balance is consistency. Try to do these exercises daily or at least a few times a week. Start with just a few minutes and gradually increase the time as you get more comfortable.

Remember, it's okay to hold onto something for support when you're starting out. Safety is the most important thing. Over time, you'll notice your balance getting better, and you'll feel more confident on your feet. So, give these exercises a try and take small steps toward better balance in your daily life.

Chapter 3

Morning Balance Awakening

A Series Of 5-Minute Morning Routines to Kickstart the Day

Feeling ready to embrace the day with a burst of positivity? You're in luck! I've put together a fantastic series of 5-minute morning routines tailored specifically for seniors. These routines are designed to be incredibly simple, so you don't have to worry about any complex moves or equipment. With just a few minutes each morning, you can set the tone for your day and infuse it with a refreshing dose of energy.

These morning routines are all about making your mornings easier and more enjoyable. They're a gentle way to kickstart your day without any overwhelming or strenuous activities. By following these straightforward routines, you'll find it easier to get out of bed, face the day with a smile, and carry that positive energy with you as you tackle whatever comes your way.

So, whether you're sipping your morning coffee, tea, or just taking a moment to enjoy the quiet, these 5-minute routines are your ticket to a brighter, more invigorated start to each day. Give them a try, and you'll soon discover how simple changes can make a big difference in how you feel throughout the day.

Deep Breathing: Let's begin with some deep breathing. Find a quiet spot to sit or lie down comfortably. Close your eyes, take a deep breath in through your nose for a count of four, hold it for a count of four, and then exhale slowly through your mouth for a count of four. Repeat this a few times. It'll help you feel more relaxed and focused.

Stretching: Next, let's get those muscles moving. Stand up, reach your arms overhead, and stretch as high as you can. Feel that wonderful stretch in your body. Now, bend down gently to touch your toes if you can. Don't worry if you can't touch them; just reach as far as you can comfortably. This helps wake up your body.

Hydration: Time for a glass of water. After a night's sleep, our bodies can be a little dehydrated. Sip on a glass of water to rehydrate yourself. It's like giving your body a refreshing morning drink.

Positive Affirmations: Think of three things you're grateful for or three positive things you want to achieve today. It could be as simple as "I'm grateful for a good night's sleep" or "I want to enjoy a nice walk today." Saying these affirmations out loud can set a positive tone for your day.

Mindful Breathing: Sit down comfortably and close your eyes. Take a moment to focus on your breath. Inhale slowly and deeply through your nose, and exhale slowly through your mouth. As you breathe, let go of any worries or tension. This helps clear your mind and prepares you for the day ahead.

Light Exercise: It's important to get your blood flowing. March in place for a minute or do some gentle leg lifts while holding onto a stable surface for support. This helps boost your energy levels and gets your body ready for the day.

Breakfast: They say breakfast is the most important meal of the day, and it's true. Grab a quick and healthy breakfast like a bowl of oatmeal, a banana, or some yogurt with berries. This will give you the fuel you need to tackle the day.

Plan Your Day: Take a moment to jot down a short to-do list for the day. Include tasks you want to accomplish and any appointments you have. Having a plan can help you stay organized and focused.

Morning Stroll: If you have a safe and pleasant outdoor area nearby, consider taking a short morning stroll. It doesn't have to be a long walk, just a few minutes to enjoy the fresh air and nature around you. If you can't go outside, even looking out the window and appreciating the morning view can be refreshing.

Smile and Be Grateful: Finally, as you finish your morning routine, take a moment to smile. It's amazing what a simple smile can do for your mood. And once again, think of something you're grateful for. Maybe it's the sunshine outside or the comfort of your home. Gratitude can set a positive tone for your day.

Remember, these routines are all about taking a few moments for yourself each morning. They're gentle, and you can adjust them to fit your comfort level. There you have it, a series of 5-minute morning routines that are easy to follow and perfect for seniors. Remember, the key is to start your day with a sense of calm and positivity. These routines can help you do just that, so go ahead and give them a try. Here's to many happy and healthy mornings ahead! Starting your day with these simple practices can make a big difference in how you feel throughout the day. So, give them a try, and here's to a great day ahead!

Focus on Balance Exercises that Promote Energy and Vitality

Today, we're going to talk about something super important: balance exercises that'll help you feel full of energy and vitality. Now, I know we're not all spring chickens anymore, but that doesn't mean we can't have a little bounce in our step, right?

So, why should we care about balance exercises? Well, first off, they can help us avoid those not-so-fun tumbles and falls. Plus, when we're balanced and steady on our feet, we feel more confident and independent. That's a win-win!

Let's dive into some simple and easy-peasy balance exercises that anyone can do. No need for fancy equipment or a personal trainer. Just find a comfy spot, and let's get started.

The One-Leg Stand: Stand up straight, find something sturdy to hold onto if you need it (like a chair or a wall), and lift one foot off the ground. Try to hold it for 10-15 seconds, then switch to the other foot. Do this a few times a day, and you'll be surprised at how your balance improves.

The Heel-to-Toe Walk: Pretend you're walking on a tightrope. Put one foot in front of the other, with your heel touching the toe of the opposite foot. Take small steps and keep your arms out to the sides for balance. It's like your own mini circus act!

The Chair Squat: This one's great for building leg strength and balance. Stand in front of a sturdy chair with your feet hip-width apart. Slowly lower your hips down like you're about to sit in the chair, then stand back up. Repeat 10-15 times.

The Tree Pose: Stand up straight and shift your weight onto one leg. Bend the other leg and place the sole of your foot against your inner thigh, calf, or ankle – wherever you're comfortable. You can use a chair or a wall for support if needed. Imagine you're a graceful tree swaying in the wind.

Marching in Place: Stand up beside your chair or use it for support. Lift your knees up, one at a time, as if you're marching in place. Try to do this for a minute or two. It's a fantastic way to get your heart rate up while working on balance.

Back Leg Raises: Hold onto a chair or the kitchen counter for support. Lift one leg straight back behind you while keeping your upper body straight. Hold for a few seconds, then lower it down. Repeat this 10-15 times for each leg. This move is excellent for strengthening your lower back and glutes.

Side Leg Raises: Again, use a chair or counter for balance. Lift one leg out to the side, keeping it straight. Hold for a moment and then lower it back down. Do 10-15 reps on each leg. This exercise helps strengthen your hips and outer thighs.

Balloon Volleyball: This one's a blast! Blow up a balloon and stand on one side of the room, and have a partner stand on the other side. Your goal? Keep the balloon from touching the ground by hitting it back and forth. It's a fun way to work on your balance and coordination while having a good laugh.

Staying active and balanced is not only good for your body but also for your mood and overall well-being. It's like a secret recipe for a happier and healthier you!

So, don't be shy; give these exercises a try, and have some fun while you're at it. Balance is the name of the game, and you've got this! Enjoy the journey to more energy and vitality. Remember, the key to these exercises is to start slowly and gradually increase the time or repetitions as you feel more comfortable. And always put safety first! If you're not sure about a particular exercise, it's a good idea to check with your healthcare provider. Some fun and easy balance exercises to help you feel more energetic and full of life. Keep at it, and before you know it, you'll be strutting your stuff with the best of them. Stay active, stay balanced, and keep that vitality flowing!

Mindfulness Techniques for a Positive Outlook

Today, let's talk about something super cool and totally chill; mindfulness techniques!

Now, you might be wondering, "What's all the buzz about mindfulness?" Well, it's like giving your brain a spa day! It's all about being in the moment, soaking up the good stuff, and letting go of the stress and worries.

Here are some easy-peasy mindfulness techniques to help you rock that positive outlook:

Breathe In, Breathe Out: Okay, let's talk about the power of your breath! This mindfulness technique is as easy as, well, breathing! Find yourself a comfy spot, whether it's a cozy chair or your favorite couch. Sit or lie down, and if you're feeling fancy, close your eyes (if not, that's cool too).

Now, here's the trick: take a deep breath in through your nose, just like you're smelling the most scrumptious batch of cookies fresh out of the oven. Imagine those warm, delightful smells wafting into your nose.

Next, slowly exhale through your mouth, like you're blowing out the candles on a birthday cake. Feel that tension and stress melting away with each breath out.

Repeat this a few times, and you'll start feeling more relaxed than a lazy Sunday afternoon. Your mind will clear up, and you'll be ready to take on whatever the day throws your way. Remember, it's all about slowing down and giving your brain a little vacation. Ah, refreshing!

Nature's Show: Who here loves the great outdoors? If you do, you're in for a treat because nature is like the world's best show, and guess what? It's free! Step outside, whether it's your backyard, a park down the street, or just your front porch, and take a moment to soak it all in. Look up at the sky; it could be a clear blue canvas or maybe it's painted with fluffy clouds.

Listen closely; hear the birds singing their hearts out? Maybe there's a gentle breeze rustling the leaves in the trees. It's like a symphony of nature's sounds.

And don't forget to use those other senses too! Take a deep breath; what scents are lingering in the air? Can you feel the warmth of the sun on your skin or the coolness of the shade under a tree? Touch the bark of a tree or the softness of a flower petal.

Nature's like a live show that never gets old. It's a reminder that the world is a beautiful place, and we're a part of it. So, take a front-row seat, breathe it all in, and let Mother Nature put on her best performance just for you.

There you have it, folks – two simple and delightful ways to embrace mindfulness and bring a little extra sunshine into your day!

Mindful Munching: Hey there, snack enthusiasts! Let's chat about something we all love munching! But this time, we're going to munch mindfully, and trust me, it's a game-changer.

Grab your favorite snack, whether it's a crunchy carrot stick or a piece of chocolate that's calling your name. Now, find a comfy spot to sit down. It could be your kitchen table or your favorite chair; wherever you feel relaxed.

Take a moment to really look at your snack. Notice the colors, the textures, and any little details. If it's a carrot, admire its vibrant orange color. If it's chocolate, check out those delightful swirls.

Now, take a bite, but don't rush it. Chew slowly and pay attention to the flavors dancing on your taste buds. Is it sweet, salty, or maybe a little bit of both? Let the taste fill your senses.

Feel the sensation of chewing and the food moving in your mouth. You're not just eating; you're experiencing every little detail of your snack.

This mindful munching isn't just about enjoying your food more; it's about being fully present in the moment and savoring the simple pleasures of life. So go ahead, munch away, and let your taste buds throw a party!

Five Senses Game: Alrighty, it's time to play the "Five Senses Game" on board, no dice, just your awesome senses! Find a comfy spot to sit or stand, wherever you're feeling super chill. Now, let's dive into your senses:

Sight: Look around and take in the sights. What colors are catching your eye? Is there something interesting on the wall, like a picture or a painting? Maybe you see a bright blue sky or some flowers in your garden. Enjoy the visual feast!

Sound: What can you hear right now? Close your eyes for a moment and listen carefully. It could be the hum of the refrigerator, birds chirping outside, or even the soft murmur of your own breathing. The world is full of sounds; let them serenade you!

Smell: Take a deep breath through your nose. What scents are wafting your way? It could be the aroma of dinner cooking in the kitchen, the freshness of your laundry, or even the fragrance of your favorite candle. Breathe it in, and let those scents paint a picture in your mind.

Touch: Pay attention to what you're touching right now. Maybe you're holding a warm cup of tea, feeling the softness of your clothes, or sitting in a comfy chair. Take a moment to appreciate the textures and sensations around you.

Taste: Is there a lingering taste in your mouth? Maybe it's from your last meal or a sip of your drink. If not, take a sip of water or a bite of a snack. Notice the taste as it spreads across your tongue. It's like a flavor adventure!

The "Five Senses Game" is all about tuning into the world around you. It's like unlocking a treasure chest of sensations that you might have missed in your busy day. So, go ahead and play this game anytime you want to feel more connected to the present moment. It's like a sensory vacation!

Body Scan: Let's talk about a super relaxing and simple mindfulness technique called the "Body Scan." Find a comfy spot to lie down, like your bed or a cozy carpet. You can even do this on a couch if that's more your style. Close your eyes and take a deep breath to start. Now, imagine a gentle spotlight shining on your toes. Yep, you're the star of the show! As that spotlight moves slowly up your body, focus your attention on each part it touches.

Start with your toes; wiggle them a bit, and then let them relax. Feel any tension melting away. Move up to your feet, your ankles, and your legs. As you go, notice any sensations; warmth, coolness, or maybe a little tingle.

Keep that spotlight moving, up through your body. Relax your belly, your chest, and your shoulders. Let go of any tightness or stress. It's like a soothing massage for your mind and body.

As the spotlight reaches your arms, your neck, and your head, take your time to release any tension you find. By the time it reaches the tippy-top of your head, you'll feel as calm as a serene lake on a peaceful day.

The "Body Scan" is like a little vacation for your body and mind. It's perfect for unwinding after a busy day or just taking a break to recharge. So, go ahead, scan away, and let the relaxation flow!

Scott Anthony

Chapter 4

Midday Balance Recharge

Quick and Discreet Balance Exercises Suitable for any Location

We've got a fun and easy-peasy topic to talk about today: balance exercises that you can do pretty much anywhere, and they won't draw too much attention. Whether you're in the comfort of your own home or out and about, these exercises are perfect for seniors who want to stay steady on their feet. No fancy gym equipment or complicated routines needed; just you and a little bit of space.

Heel-To-Toe Walk: This exercise is all about mastering balance while taking measured steps. Start by standing up straight with your feet together. Imagine you're on a tightrope, and to mimic that, place one foot directly in front of the other, so your heel touches the toes of your other foot. Keep your arms relaxed by your sides or extend them out to the sides for better balance. Now, take slow, deliberate steps, making sure your heel touches the toes of the foot in front of it with each step. Try to keep your gaze fixed ahead of you, not down at your feet. This exercise mimics the precision required for maintaining balance, just like a tightrope walker.

Kitchen Counter Shuffle: This one is like a little dance routine you can do in your kitchen. Stand sideways to your kitchen counter, lightly holding onto it for support. Your feet should be hip-width apart. Start by taking small, controlled steps to the side while keeping your hands on the counter. It's like a slow-motion sidestep. Once you reach the end of the counter, turn around and shuffle back the other way. The kitchen counter is your trusty partner in this dance, and it provides a bit of support if you need it. This exercise helps improve your lateral balance, which is essential for avoiding slips and falls.

Wall Angels: For this exercise, you'll need a flat wall as your workout buddy. Stand with your back against the wall and your feet about hip-width apart. Begin by slowly raising both of your arms up the wall as high as you comfortably can. Imagine you're drawing angel wings on the wall with your fingertips. Keep your palms facing forward as you raise your arms. Then, lower your arms back down in a controlled manner. The wall provides support while you work on your balance, and this exercise helps improve your posture as well as shoulder and upper back strength.

Balance on One Foot While Brushing Your Teeth: Here's a fantastic way to make the most of your morning routine. While brushing your teeth, make sure to brace yourself or hold onto something as you stand on one foot. It's like a balancing act while you maintain your oral hygiene! Start by lifting one foot slightly off the ground and keeping it steady as you brush your teeth. After a minute or two, switch to the other foot. This exercise challenges your balance in a real-life situation and helps strengthen your leg muscles and core. Remember, it's perfectly okay to use a nearby wall or countertop for support when you're starting these exercises, and over time, you can gradually reduce your reliance on them as your balance improves. These simple yet effective exercises can help you stay steady on your feet and prevent falls, making daily life safer and more enjoyable. So go ahead, give them a try, and have fun while you're at it

Stress-Relief Practices to Combat Midday Tension

Feeling a bit stressed in the middle of the day? Don't worry, you're not alone in this! It happens to the best of us, especially when life gets a bit hectic and we're juggling a hundred things at once. But guess what? There are some easy-peasy ways to kick that midday tension to the curb, and you don't need a PhD in relaxation to do them. So, put your worries aside for a moment, and let's have a friendly chat about some stress-relief practices that are as simple and comforting as enjoying a cup of tea on a rainy afternoon.

Breathe It Out: Picture this: stress starts tiptoeing into your day like an unwelcome guest, and suddenly, you realize you've forgotten how to breathe. It happens to the best of us. The good news is, you can kick stress to the curb with a simple but powerful technique - deep breathing.

Find a quiet spot to sit down, even if it's just for a few moments. Close your eyes if you feel comfortable doing so. Now, take a deep breath in through your nose, counting to four as you do. Feel your chest and belly rise as you fill your lungs with fresh air.

Then, exhale gently through your mouth, counting to six this time. Let go of all that tension and worries with your breath. As you repeat this process a few times, you'll start to notice some magical things happening.

First, your racing thoughts will quiet down, like a bustling street settling into a peaceful evening. Second, your heart rate will slow down, like a fast-paced song transitioning into a soothing lullaby. And guess what? You'll start to feel more relaxed and centered, like you're sitting in the eye of a storm, untouched by the chaos around you.

This simple breathing exercise is like a reset button for your mind and body. It reminds you that you have the power to control stress, just by taking a few moments to breathe deeply and intentionally. So, the next time stress sneaks up on you, remember to breathe it out. It's your secret weapon for finding calm in the midst of chaos.

Stretch It Out: Sitting at your desk or in front of the TV for too long can make you feel like a human pretzel with stiff muscles. But fear not, because there's a simple trick to loosen up and recharge your body: stretching!

Imagine yourself as a sunflower reaching for the sun. Stand up and stretch your arms high above your head. Reach for the sky as if you're trying to touch the clouds. Feel your spine lengthen and take a deep breath. It's like waking up your body from a long nap.

Now, slowly, like a graceful willow in the wind, bend forward at your waist. Let your arms dangle towards your toes or as far as you comfortably can. Don't push too hard; just go where your body allows. Feel the tension in your muscles ease away as you hold the stretch for a few seconds.

This simple stretch is like opening the curtains to let the sunshine in. It increases blood flow, sending a wave of refreshment to every corner of your body. Muscle tension surrenders, and you'll find yourself with an instant energy boost. It's like hitting the reset button for your day, and your body will thank you with a sigh of relief. So, whenever you're feeling a bit sluggish or stressed, take a moment to stretch it out and let the good vibes flow. Your body will thank you for it!

Nature Break: When life's pressures start piling up, and you're stuck indoors, there's something truly magical about taking a moment to step outside. Nature has this incredible power to calm your racing mind and soothe your soul.

All you need to do is open that door, breathe in that fresh air, and let the world outside work its wonders. Take a short walk, even if it's just around your garden or a nearby park. As you stroll, look at the trees swaying gently in the breeze. Listen to the birds chirping and the leaves rustling. It's like a mini mental vacation that costs nothing and yet offers priceless benefits.

You'll find that this brief connection with nature can help you hit the reset button on your day. When you return to your tasks, you'll do so with a clearer mind, a lighter heart, and a renewed sense of purpose. Nature has this beautiful way of reminding us to slow down, take a moment, and appreciate the simple and calming beauty that surrounds us every day.

Caffeine Control: Ah, the beloved cup of coffee in the morning - it's like a warm hug for your brain, isn't it? But here's the thing: while a little caffeine can be your buddy, too much can turn it into a jittery, heart-pounding frenemy. That's where caffeine control comes into play.

You see, caffeine is like a rollercoaster ride for your nerves. It gives you a quick burst of energy, but then it can leave you feeling anxious and shaky. So, here's a simple trick to keep your nerves steady, especially in the afternoon.

Consider switching things up. Instead of reaching for that second (or third) cup of coffee, opt for something gentler on your nerves. Herbal tea is a fantastic choice. There are so many flavors to explore, from soothing chamomile to refreshing peppermint. It's like giving your taste buds a little adventure without the caffeine-induced drama.

Tech Timeout: We're all guilty of spending too much time on our phones or computers. Give yourself a break by putting your devices away for a little while. This will help you disconnect from the constant stream of information and notifications, giving your mind a chance to recharge.

Positive Vibes: Think of a happy memory or something that brings a smile to your face. It could be a hilarious moment with friends or a beautiful sunset you witnessed. Let your mind wander to that place, and you'll find that your mood lifts as you remember the good things in life.

Snack Smart: When hunger strikes, it can make stress feel even worse. Keep a healthy snack on hand, like a banana or a small handful of nuts. These snacks provide a quick energy boost and help stabilize your blood sugar levels, keeping those hangry feelings at bay.

Music Magic: Music has a remarkable ability to influence our mood. Put on your favorite song or create a playlist of calming tunes. Close your eyes and let the music transport you to a more relaxed state of mind. It's like a mini escape from the stress of the day.

Remember, these stress-relief practices are your personal toolbox of tranquility. You can pick and choose which ones work best for you or combine them to create your own perfect stress-busting routine. The key is to take it slow, be kind to yourself, and find the techniques that make your midday tension a thing of the past.

Breathing Exercises for Relaxation and Focus

We're going to talk about something super easy and incredibly helpful for keeping calm and staying focused: breathing exercises. Yup, you heard that right; just breathing can work wonders! So, let's dive in.

Deep Belly Breathing: Deep belly breathing is a simple yet powerful technique to help you relax and regain focus. Find a comfortable place to sit or lie down. Close your eyes if it feels comfortable. Now, take a slow, deep breath in through your nose, allowing your belly to expand as you breathe in, almost like a balloon inflating. Count to four in your mind as you do this.

After you've inhaled deeply, exhale slowly and steadily through your mouth for another count of four. This is like letting the air out of that balloon. Feel your body relax as you release your breath. Repeat this deep belly breathing exercise a few times.

The magic of this exercise is that it shifts your body from the "fight or flight" mode to "rest and digest." It's like a reset button for your nervous system, reducing stress and increasing your overall sense of calm.

Box Breathing: Box breathing is a simple and effective technique that can help you manage stress and stay focused. It's a technique that was created by the Navy Seals – you can imagine the stress they must be under. Start by finding a comfortable position, either sitting or lying down, and close your eyes if it feels right for you.

Imagine drawing a square or a box with your breath. Inhale slowly and deeply through your nose for a count of four. Then, hold your breath for another count of four. Now, exhale gently and completely through your mouth for another count of four. Finally, pause and hold your breath again for a count of four.

Repeat this box pattern a few times, and you'll notice how it calms your mind and brings you into the present moment. Box breathing is like a mental reset button, helping you regain control over your thoughts and emotions.

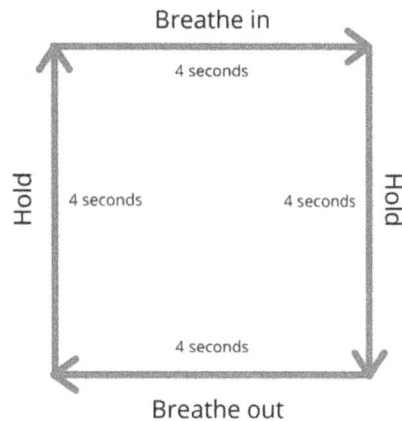

```
                    Breathe in
              ┌─────────────────────┐
              │      4 seconds      │
              │                     │
        Hold  │ 4 seconds  4 seconds│  Hold
              │                     │
              │      4 seconds      │
              └─────────────────────┘
                   Breathe out
```

4-7-8 Breathing: The 4-7-8 breathing technique is a simple and effective way to relax your body and mind. To start, find a quiet and comfortable place to sit or lie down. Close your eyes if it feels comfortable.

Begin by taking a slow, deep breath in through your nose for a count of four. Feel your lungs fill with air as you do this. After inhaling, hold your breath for a count of seven. This pause allows your body to absorb oxygen and calm your nervous system.

Next, exhale slowly and completely through your mouth for a count of eight. As you breathe out, imagine releasing tension and stress with each breath. This technique can be repeated a few times to help you feel more relaxed and centered.

4-7-8 breathing is like a natural tranquilizer for your body and mind. It's a handy tool to have in your relaxation toolkit.

Alternate Nostril Breathing: Alternate nostril breathing may sound complex, but it's a straightforward technique to balance your energy and calm your mind. Find a comfortable place to sit with your spine straight, and you can rest your left hand on your lap.

Using your right thumb and ring finger, gently block off one nostril while you breathe in through the other nostril. Inhale slowly and deeply, counting to four as you do.

Now, switch sides. Close off the nostril you just breathed in through and exhale through the other nostril for a count of four. Continue this alternating pattern, inhaling and exhaling through each nostril for a few cycles.

Alternate nostril breathing helps balance the left and right sides of your brain and promotes a sense of calm and focus. It's like a yoga session for your nose!

Beach Breathing: Beach breathing is a delightful visualization technique that can transport you to a serene mental oasis. Close your eyes and imagine yourself at the beach, listening to the soothing sound of waves crashing. As you breathe in through your nose, envision taking in the fresh ocean air. Inhale slowly, counting to four, and imagine the salty breeze filling your lungs.

Now, exhale through your mouth for a count of four, as if you're gently blowing out a sandcastle on the shore. Feel the stress and worries melting away with each exhalation.

Repeat this beach breathing exercise for a few minutes, and you'll find yourself feeling more relaxed, as if you've taken a mini-vacation for your mind. It's like bringing a piece of the beach into your daily life, wherever you are.

Encouragement for Mindful Eating During Lunch

Now we're going to chat about something that's pretty important but often overlooked: mindful eating during lunch. Now, I know we're all busy bees, and sometimes it's tempting to just grab a quick bite and move on with our day. But taking a moment to eat mindfully can actually do wonders for our health and well-being.

So, what's mindful eating, you ask? Well, it's all about paying full attention to your food and how you eat it. It's not just shoveling it in while you're watching TV or scrolling through your phone. Nope, it's about savoring each bite, appreciating the flavors, and listening to your body.

Here are a few reasons why mindful eating during lunch can be a game-changer:

Encouragement For Mindful Eating During Lunch: We're going to chat about something that's pretty important but often overlooked: mindful eating during lunch. Now, I know we're all busy bees, and sometimes it's tempting to just grab a quick bite and move on with our day. But taking a moment to eat mindfully can actually do wonders for our health and well-being.

So, what's mindful eating, you ask? Well, it's all about paying full attention to your food and how you eat it. It's not just shoveling it in while you're watching TV or scrolling through your phone. Nope, it's about savoring each bite, appreciating the flavors, and listening to your body.

Here are a few reasons why mindful eating during lunch can be a game-changer:

1. Digestion: When you're eating in a rush or while distracted, your body might not be prepared to digest the food properly. This can lead to tummy troubles. But when you eat mindfully, you're sending a signal to your body that it's time to start the digestion process, which can help prevent discomfort.

2. Portion Control: Mindful eating helps you recognize when you're full. That means you're less likely to overeat and feel stuffed after lunch. It's a great way to keep those extra calories in check.

3. Enjoyment: Eating should be an enjoyable experience, not just a task to check off your to-do list. When you savor each bite, you'll find that your meals become more satisfying, and you appreciate the taste of your food even more.

Now, let's talk about some simple tips to get you started on your mindful eating journey:

- **Chew Slowly:** Take your time with each bite. Chewing slowly not only helps with digestion but also allows you to fully taste and enjoy your food.

- **Appreciate the Colors and Textures:** Take a moment to look at your meal. Notice the colors, textures, and aromas. It's like a little food adventure!

- **Listen to Your Body**: Pay attention to your hunger and fullness cues. Stop eating when you're satisfied, not when your plate is empty.

- **Stay Hydrated:** Sometimes, our bodies confuse thirst with hunger. So, make sure to have a glass of water before your meal to help gauge your true hunger.

Remember, there's no need to be perfect at this right away. It's all about progress, not perfection. So, take small steps toward more mindful eating during lunch, and you'll likely start noticing some positive changes in how you feel. Enjoy your meals, savor the flavors, and treat yourself to a little self-care during lunchtime. You deserve it!

Encouragement For Mindful Eating During Lunch: Now that we've covered the basics, let's dive a bit deeper into why being mindful during lunchtime is so beneficial and how you can make it a daily habit. Weight Management: Mindful eating can help you manage your weight more effectively. By paying attention to your body's signals, you're less likely to overindulge in high-calorie, low-nutrition foods. It's a great way to maintain a healthy weight without feeling like you're constantly dieting.

Lunchtime can be a welcome break from a busy day. Use it as an opportunity to de-stress and unwind. When you're fully present in the moment, you can savor your meal and let go of worries, even if it's just for a little while. Improved Digestion Eating mindfully promotes better digestion. Your body can focus on breaking down and absorbing nutrients more efficiently when it's not distracted by other activities or stress.

Mind-Body Connection: Being mindful of what you eat helps you connect with your body's needs and preferences. You might discover that certain foods make you feel great, while others leave you sluggish. This awareness can guide your food choices in the long run. Gratitude: Taking a moment to appreciate your meal can foster gratitude. Think about where your food came from, the effort that went into preparing it, and the nourishment it provides. It's a simple practice that can boost your overall well-being.

Now, let's wrap things up with a few more tips to help you make mindful eating a part of your daily routine:

- Set the Mood: Create a pleasant atmosphere for your meal. Use nice tableware, light a candle, or play some soothing music. It's all about making lunchtime a special occasion.

- Start Small: If you're new to mindful eating, don't overwhelm yourself. Begin with one meal a day, like lunch, and gradually incorporate it into your routine.

- Practice Gratitude: Before you dig in, take a moment to express gratitude for your food. It can be a simple "thank you" for the nourishment it provides.

- Share the Experience: If you can, enjoy lunch with friends or family. Sharing a meal can enhance the experience and encourage mindful eating.

There's no need to be perfect at this right away. It's all about progress, not perfection. So, take small steps toward more mindful eating during lunch, and you'll likely start noticing some positive changes in how you feel. Enjoy your meals, savor the flavors, and treat yourself to a little self-care during lunchtime. You deserve it! So, there you have it, folks! Mindful eating during lunch is a simple yet powerful way to improve your health and well-being. Give it a try, and don't forget to enjoy your food; it's one of life's greatest pleasures.

Scott Anthony

Chapter 5

Evening Balance Tranquillity

Gentle Exercises to Wind Down and Prepare for a Restful Night

If you're like me and sometimes find it a bit tricky to wind down before bed, I've got some easy-peasy exercises that might just do the trick. We're talking gentle moves that won't require you to be a contortionist or a fitness guru. These are perfect for seniors or anyone looking to relax and get a good night's sleep.

Neck Rolls: Neck rolls are a simple and effective way to relax your neck muscles before bedtime. Begin by sitting or standing up straight, making sure your back is comfortably aligned. Gently tilt your head to one side, bringing your ear towards your shoulder. It's like you're trying to touch your ear to your shoulder, but don't force it.

Once you feel a gentle stretch, start rolling your head in a slow, circular motion, taking care not to rush. Breathe deeply and naturally as you do this. Roll your head a few times in one direction and then switch to the other side. You should feel tension and stress melting away from your neck and shoulders.

Remember not to push your head too far or too fast, as this is all about relaxation. Go at your own pace, and if you encounter any pain or discomfort, stop immediately. It's all about feeling good and preparing your body for a restful night's sleep.

Shoulder Shrugs: Shoulder shrugs are fantastic for releasing tension in your shoulders, which can build up during the day. To do this simple exercise, sit or stand up straight with your arms relaxed at your sides. Take a deep breath in, and as you exhale, raise your shoulders up towards your ears.

Hold this raised position for a few seconds to really feel the stretch, and then slowly release your shoulders as you exhale again. You can repeat this a few times, and with each shrug, imagine letting go of any stress or worries that might be weighing you down.

Remember to keep it gentle; there's no need to force your shoulders upwards. The idea here is to relax and unwind, preparing your body for a peaceful night's sleep.

Deep Breathing: Deep breathing is a powerful tool for relaxation. Find a comfortable sitting or lying position, close your eyes, and take a moment to center yourself. Inhale slowly through your nose, counting to four in your mind. Feel your chest and abdomen expand as you breathe in.

Hold your breath for a count of four, and then exhale slowly and steadily through your mouth, counting to six this time. As you exhale, imagine all the tension and stress leaving your body with each breath.

Repeat this deep breathing exercise for a few cycles. It's like a natural tranquilizer that calms your nervous system and prepares you for a peaceful night's sleep.

Gentle Leg Stretches: Gentle leg stretches can help relax your leg muscles, which can be especially beneficial if you've been on your feet all day. Sit on the edge of your bed or a chair with your back straight.

Extend one leg out in front of you and flex your toes towards your nose. You should feel a gentle stretch along the back of your leg. Hold this position for a few seconds, making sure it's comfortable, and then relax your leg.

Switch to the other leg and repeat the stretch. This exercise is a soothing way to release tension in your legs and prepare your body for a restful night's sleep.

Bedtime Toe Taps: Bedtime toe taps are a simple and effective way to release any remaining tension and signal to your body that it's time to wind down. Sit comfortably on your bed or a chair and rest your feet on the floor.

Now, gently tap your toes on the floor for about a minute. It's like a rhythmic, soothing motion that encourages relaxation. Feel the tension in your feet and legs melt away as you tap.

This exercise is a gentle way to help you transition from the busyness of the day to a state of calm, perfect for a restful night's sleep.

Mindful Meditation: Mindful meditation is a peaceful practice that can prepare your mind and body for sleep. Find a quiet and comfortable spot to sit or lie down. Close your eyes and take a moment to let go of any distractions.

Focus your attention on your breathing. Inhale slowly and deeply through your nose, allowing your lungs to fill with air. As you exhale through your mouth, let go of any tension or racing thoughts.

Picture a tranquil place in your mind, like a calm beach, a serene forest, or your favorite peaceful spot. Imagine yourself there, feeling completely relaxed and at ease.

Continue this practice for a few minutes, allowing your mind to unwind and your body to prepare for a restful night's sleep.

Progressive Muscle Relaxation: Progressive muscle relaxation is a technique that can help you release tension throughout your body. Find a comfortable lying position in your bed.

Start with your toes. Tense the muscles in your toes for a few seconds, then release. Feel the relaxation flow through your toes.

Move on to your calf muscles. Tense them for a moment and then release. Continue this pattern, working your way up through your legs, torso, arms, and finally, your face and neck.

With each muscle group you tense and release, imagine any stress or tension melting away, leaving your body feeling light and relaxed. This exercise is an excellent way to prepare your body for a restful night's sleep.

Remember, these exercises are all about relaxation, not pushing your body to its limits. Take your time, go at your own pace, and enjoy the journey towards a restful night's sleep. Sweet dreams!

Mindfulness Meditation for Relaxation and Emotional Balance

Sure thing! Let's break down mindfulness meditation for relaxation and emotional balance in a simple and easy-to-understand way.

Have you ever heard of mindfulness meditation? It might sound a bit fancy, but don't worry, it's actually a super simple and helpful practice for calming your mind and finding balance in your emotions.

Okay, let's get started. Imagine this: You're sitting in a comfy chair, or maybe even just on your bed. You don't need any special equipment or fancy yoga poses for this. Just you, yourself, and a few moments of peace.

First, take a few deep breaths. Inhale slowly through your nose, and then exhale gently through your mouth. Feel the air going in and out. This is the first step in mindfulness meditation - focusing on your breath.

Now, let's talk about thoughts. Our minds are like busy bees, always buzzing around with thoughts about yesterday, today, or tomorrow. And that's okay! But sometimes, these thoughts can make us feel a bit overwhelmed or stressed.

Here's where mindfulness comes in. Instead of chasing those thoughts, imagine you're watching clouds in the sky. When a thought comes by, just acknowledge it like, "Hey there, thought!" and let it float away, like a cloud moving across the sky. No need to judge or hold onto it.

Back to your breath. Focus on the sensation of your breath as it goes in and out. Feel the rise and fall of your chest or the coolness of the air in your nose. This helps anchor you in the present moment, away from the worries of the past or future.

If your mind starts wandering (and it will, that's totally normal!), gently bring your attention back to your breath. It's like training a puppy; you guide it back when it wanders off. Now, let's talk about emotions. Sometimes, we feel happy, sad, anxious, or angry. It's all part of being human. Mindfulness helps us notice these emotions without getting swept away by them. You can say, "Ah, there's that feeling of sadness," and just observe it without judgment.

As you practice this mindfulness meditation, you'll start to notice that you can choose how you respond to your thoughts and emotions. It's like having a superpower - the power to stay calm and centered even when life gets a little crazy.

Remember, there's no right or wrong way to do this. You're not trying to "empty" your mind or become a meditation guru. It's all about being kind to yourself and finding a little peace in your day.

So, whether you're feeling stressed, anxious, or just want a moment to relax, give mindfulness meditation a try. It's like a mini-vacation for your mind, and you deserve it

Absolutely, let's keep going on our journey to mindfulness meditation for relaxation and emotional balance. We're going to explore a few more tips and tricks that will make this practice even more accessible and enjoyable.

★ **Start Small:** You don't need to meditate for hours on end. Even just a few minutes a day can make a big difference. Gradually, you can increase the time as you get more comfortable with the practice.

★ **Create a Peaceful Space:** Find a quiet spot where you won't be disturbed. Maybe it's your favorite chair, a cozy corner, or a peaceful park bench. Make it your special place to meditate.

★ **Use Guided Meditations:** If you're not sure where to start, there are plenty of guided meditations available online. These are like having a friendly voice gently lead you through the process, which can be especially helpful for beginners.

★ **Be Patient with Yourself:** Don't expect instant results. Mindfulness meditation is a bit like planting seeds; you won't see the flowers right away. Over time, though, you'll notice positive changes in your mood and how you handle stress.

★ **Incorporate Mindfulness into Daily Life:** You don't have to meditate only while sitting still. You can practice mindfulness while doing everyday activities like walking, eating, or even washing dishes. Just pay attention to what you're doing at that moment.

★ **Stay Open-Minded:** Your experience with mindfulness meditation might vary from day to day. Some days, your mind might be calm as a lake; other days, it might feel like a stormy sea. That's okay! Accept whatever comes up during your practice without judgment.

★ **Be Consistent:** Like any skill, mindfulness gets better with practice. Try to incorporate it into your daily routine, and you'll find that it becomes more natural over time.

★ **Share the Practice:** If you have a friend or family member who might benefit from mindfulness, consider sharing your experience with them. You can even meditate together. It's a wonderful way to connect and support each other.

Remember, mindfulness meditation is a simple and effective way to bring more peace and balance into your life. It's all about taking a moment to pause, breathe, and be kind to yourself. So, go ahead, give it a try, and see how it can work wonders for your relaxation and emotional well-being.

Creating a Peaceful Bedtime Routine

Set a Regular Bedtime: The key to a peaceful bedtime routine is consistency. Choose a bedtime that works for you and try to stick to it every night. Our bodies love routines, and having a consistent bedtime helps train your internal sleep clock. It's like telling your body, "Hey, it's time to wind down." When you go to bed at the same time each night, your body learns when to start releasing sleep-inducing hormones, making it easier to fall asleep and wake up feeling refreshed.

Turn Off Those Screens: In today's digital age, we're surrounded by screens, but they can interfere with our sleep. The blue light emitted by phones, tablets, and TVs tells your brain to stay awake. To create a peaceful bedtime routine, try to switch off these gadgets at least an hour before bed. Instead of staring at screens, consider reading a physical book, listening to calming music, or engaging in a quiet, screen-free activity that relaxes your mind.

Create a Cozy Atmosphere: Transform your bedroom into a haven of tranquility. Soft lighting, plush pillows, and a warm, comfortable blanket can work wonders. A clutter-free room can also help ease your mind, promoting a sense of serenity and calm. Your bedroom should be a place where you can escape the stresses of the day and feel at ease as you prepare for a restful night's sleep.

Unwind with Calm Activities: As bedtime approaches, it's essential to unwind and let go of the day's stress. Engage in activities that promote relaxation, such as light stretching or yoga, meditating, or practicing deep breathing exercises. These activities help calm your nervous system and signal to your body that it's time to relax and prepare for sleep. Consider creating a bedtime routine that includes these calming practices to make your transition to sleep smoother.

Watch Your Snacking: Your choice of evening snacks can impact your sleep quality. Consuming a heavy meal right before bed might lead to discomfort and restlessness. Instead, opt for a light, healthy snack like a banana, a small bowl of cereal, or a cup of herbal tea. These choices can provide a sense of satisfaction without overloading your digestive system, making it easier to settle into a peaceful slumber.

Limit Caffeine and Alcohol: What you consume in the evening can significantly affect your sleep. Caffeine and alcohol are two culprits that can disrupt your slumber. Try to avoid these substances too close to bedtime. Caffeine, found in coffee, tea, and some sodas, is a stimulant that can keep you awake, so it's a good idea to enjoy your last cup of coffee earlier in the day. Alcohol might make you feel drowsy initially, but it can lead to fragmented sleep and wake you up during the night. Consider switching to a soothing herbal tea or a warm glass of milk before bed for a more restful sleep.

Stay Hydrated (But Not Too Much): Proper hydration is essential for overall health, but drinking too much water right before bed can lead to nighttime trips to the bathroom. To balance hydration with uninterrupted sleep, sip on water throughout the day and try to reduce your intake in the hours leading up to bedtime. This way, you'll stay comfortably hydrated without disturbances during the night.

Stick to Your Routine: Once you've established a bedtime routine that helps you relax and prepare for sleep, it's crucial to stick with it consistently. Your body loves patterns and will respond positively to a regular routine. Over time, your body will become accustomed to your bedtime cues, making it easier to fall asleep and wake up feeling refreshed. If you occasionally deviate from your routine, don't worry; just get back on track as soon as possible.

Be Patient: Sometimes, sleep can be a bit elusive, even when you've followed your bedtime routine diligently. If you find yourself lying awake in bed, try not to stress about it. Worrying about sleep can make it even harder to fall asleep. Instead, get up and do something calming and relaxing for a short while, like reading a few pages of a book or practicing gentle stretches. Then, when you feel sleepy again, return to bed and give it another try.

Get Some Sunshine: Exposure to natural light during the day plays a crucial role in regulating your sleep-wake cycle. Spending time outside, even if it's just for a short walk, can help reinforce your body's internal clock. The sunlight helps your body distinguish between day and night, making it easier to feel awake during the day and sleepy at night. So, try to get a dose of sunshine during the day to enhance the effectiveness of your bedtime routine.

In summary, creating a peaceful bedtime routine is about cultivating habits that promote relaxation and signal to your body that it's time to wind down. These simple steps can make a world of difference in your sleep quality, leaving you feeling more rested and rejuvenated each morning. Sweet dreams and restful nights await!

Creating a peaceful bedtime routine is all about prioritizing your sleep and well-being. It's a personal journey where you can discover what works best for you. By following these simple steps, you can establish a routine that promotes restful nights and ensures you wake up feeling refreshed and ready to take on a new day. Sweet dreams!

Visualizations to Enhance Sleep Quality

The Beach Sunset: Envisioning a beach at sunset is like taking a mental vacation. As you sit on the shore, feel the warmth of the sand against your skin and the gentle sea breeze. Imagine the waves lapping at the shoreline, each one carrying away your worries. The changing colors of the sky, from vibrant oranges to soothing purples, signal the transition from a busy day to a tranquil night. Embrace the feeling of relaxation and peace that washes over you, and let it prepare you for a restful night's sleep.

Starry Night Sky: Gazing at a starry night sky is a timeless practice for calming the mind. As you lay under the celestial canvas, mentally count the stars, one by one. The infinite expanse of the universe puts your worries into perspective, reminding you of the vastness of existence. With each counted star, you release tension, allowing your body to become heavier and more at ease. The calming rhythm of this visualization can gently guide you into a deep slumber.

Cloud Drifting: Picture yourself in an open sky with fluffy white clouds. Each cloud represents a worry or a stressful thought. As you watch these clouds drift away from you, they vanish into the distance. The clearing sky symbolizes the clearing of your mind. This visualization encourages you to let go of troubling thoughts and embrace a sense of mental clarity and relaxation, ideal for falling asleep peacefully.

The Forest Walk: In the forest, you embark on a soothing journey. Visualize yourself walking along a quiet forest path, surrounded by towering trees. The rustling leaves and chirping birds provide a tranquil soundtrack. Feel the earthy ground beneath your feet, connecting you with nature's calming energy. With each step, release tension and worries, allowing them to dissolve into the natural world around you. This visualization grounds you in the present moment and encourages a sense of serenity.

Breathing Color: Close your eyes and focus on your breath. Inhale slowly and visualize inhaling a calming color, such as soft blue or lavender. As you exhale, imagine releasing any stress or tension as a contrasting color, like gray or black. With each breath, your body fills with your chosen calming color, promoting relaxation. This visualization combines the power of deep, intentional breathing with the soothing influence of color therapy, making it an effective tool for achieving restful sleep.

Floating on a Calm Lake: Imagine yourself on a small boat, gently floating in the middle of a serene lake. Feel the slight rocking of the boat as you drift on the tranquil waters. Listen to the soothing sounds of nature around you—the chirping of crickets, the rustling of leaves, or the distant call of a night bird. As you float, let go of any worries or thoughts, allowing them to drift away like ripples on the water's surface. This visualization transports you to a place of peace and stillness, guiding you toward a tranquil night's rest.

Warm Candlelight: Create a mental image of a cozy room bathed in the soft, warm glow of candlelight. Imagine the flickering flames casting soothing shadows on the walls. Focus your attention on the gentle, rhythmic dance of the candle flames. The soft, ambient light creates a sense of calm and comfort. Let the tranquil atmosphere of this visualization envelop you, helping you release tension and ease into a peaceful sleep.

Incorporating these visualizations into your bedtime routine can transform your sleep experience. Whether you prefer the calming beach, the vast night sky, or any of the other scenarios, these mental journeys can help you unwind, de-stress, and prepare your mind and body for a night of deep and restorative sleep. Sweet dreams await!

Scott Anthony

Chapter 6

Weekly Balance Routines

Longer Weekly Routines for a Deeper Balance Practice

If you're looking to take your balance practice to the next level, you've come to the right place. We're going to chat about some longer weekly routines that can help you find your inner Zen and improve your balance, all while keeping things nice and relaxed.

❖ **Start Slow and Steady:** Remember, Rome wasn't built in a day, and neither is your balance. Start your weekly routine with some easy-peasy warm-up exercises. Stand up straight and try holding onto a sturdy chair for support if you need it. Slowly shift your weight from one foot to the other, feeling the muscles in your legs working. Do this for about 5 minutes, and you're off to a great start!

❖ **The Daily Balancing Act:** Try to dedicate a few minutes each day to balance exercises. This can be as simple as standing on one leg while you brush your teeth or do the dishes. Hold on to a countertop or a wall if needed. It's all about building those balanced muscles little by little.

❖ **Stretch It Out:** Flexibility plays a big role in balance. Incorporate some gentle stretching into your routine. Reach for the stars and touch your toes, but don't push yourself too hard. Stretching should feel good, not painful.

❖ **Challenge Yourself Weekly:** As you start feeling more confident, challenge yourself a bit more each week. Try standing on one leg without holding onto anything for a few seconds longer or close your eyes while doing it. Just be sure to do this in a safe environment.

❖ **Mindfulness Meditation:** Balance isn't just about your body; it's also about your mind. Try some mindfulness meditation to stay calm and focused. It can help you connect with your inner self and find your center.

Tracking Progress and Adjusting Goals.

Setting Clear Goals: Imagine you're planning a road trip. Before hitting the road, you need to know where you want to go, right? Well, setting clear goals is just like picking your destination. It's about figuring out what you want to achieve. Maybe it's learning a new recipe, saving up for a vacation, or even planting a garden. The important thing is to make your goals specific and meaningful to you.

Keeping It Simple: Now, let's talk about keeping it simple. Imagine you're juggling balls. If you try to juggle too many at once, you might drop them all. It's the same with goals. If you have too many goals, it can get confusing and overwhelming. Start with just one or two goals at a time. It makes it easier to focus and track your progress.

Measuring Progress: Think of measuring progress like checking your map during your road trip. You want to see how far you've come and how much farther you need to go. For your goals, it means keeping a record. If your goal is to exercise more, write down what you did each day; maybe you walked for 15 minutes or did some stretches. If it's saving money, keep track of how much you save each week. This way, you can see the steps you're taking toward your goal.

Celebrating Small Wins: Imagine you're climbing a big mountain. It's a tough journey, but as you go, you come across some beautiful flowers. These are like the small wins on your way to your goal. Don't forget to enjoy them! When you achieve something, no matter how small, give yourself a pat on the back. It keeps you motivated and makes the journey more enjoyable.

Staying Flexible: Life can be unpredictable, just like the weather on your road trip. Sometimes, you might encounter rain or detours. Similarly, in your journey toward your goals, things might change. You might realize you need more time, or you might find a better way to reach your goal. It's okay to adjust your plans. Being flexible is a strength, not a weakness.

Asking for Support: Imagine you're not traveling alone but with friends or family. They can help you if you get lost or need a hand. Well, in your goal journey, it's okay to ask for help too. Share your goals with loved ones, and they can cheer you on and offer guidance when needed. It's like having co-pilots on your journey.

Reflecting and Adjusting: Picture yourself taking breaks during your road trip to look at the map and decide if you need to change your route. Similarly, from time to time, take a break to think about your goals. Are you making progress? Are your goals still making you happy? If not, it's okay to adjust them. Goals are meant to serve you, not the other way around.

So, tracking progress and adjusting goals is like taking a journey. You have your destination (goals), your map (tracking progress), and the flexibility to adapt along the way. Just remember, every step you take gets you closer to where you want to be. Enjoy the journey and keep moving forward!

Celebrating Successes and Maintaining Motivation

Alright, let's talk about something that makes our journey towards our goals even more enjoyable, celebrating our successes and keeping that motivation going strong.

Celebrate Small Victories: Think of achieving your goals like climbing a mountain. Along the way, there are smaller hills and beautiful vistas. These are like the small successes you achieve on your journey. Did you finish a chapter of a book? Complete a workout? Save a little extra money? Celebrate these wins! It could be as simple as treating yourself to a favorite snack or watching your favorite show.

Acknowledge Progress: Just like a progress bar on your computer shows how far a file has downloaded, you need to acknowledge how far you've come. Take a moment to look back at where you started and appreciate the progress you've made. This reflection can be a great motivator because it shows that you're moving forward.

Set Milestones: Imagine your goal is a long road trip. Along the way, you could plan some stops to rest and enjoy the scenery. These are like milestones in your journey. Divide your big goal into smaller, achievable parts. When you reach these milestones, reward yourself. It's like having mini-celebrations on your way to the ultimate goal.

Share Your Achievements: Remember the excitement of sharing vacation photos with friends? Well, sharing your achievements with others can create a similar feeling of joy. Share your progress and successes with friends and family. They can cheer you on and celebrate with you. Their support can be a powerful motivator.

Stay Positive: Sometimes, the road gets bumpy, just like life can throw challenges your way. But staying positive is like having a sturdy car that can handle those bumps. Focus on what you've achieved and the progress you've made, even if it's small. A positive mindset can keep your motivation high.

Visualize Success: Imagine your goal is reaching a beautiful beach. Picture yourself there, feeling the warm sand between your toes and hearing the ocean waves. Visualization can be a powerful tool. Close your eyes and imagine yourself successfully achieving your goal. It can help keep your motivation alive.

Adapt and Learn: Remember, setbacks can happen. Think of them as detours on your journey, not roadblocks. Learn from your setbacks and adjust your plans as needed. It's all part of the adventure.

Stay Inspired: Just like looking at travel magazines can inspire you to plan your next trip, stay inspired by looking at what others have achieved. Read success stories or watch motivational videos related to your goal. It can reignite your motivation.

In the end, celebrating your successes and maintaining motivation is like fueling your journey. It's the pep talk, the energy boost, and the fun part of working towards your goals. So, don't forget to pat yourself on the back, keep your spirits high, and enjoy the ride! You've got this!

Engaging in Group Routines for Community Support

Hey there! Let's chat about something wonderful that can bring people together and create a strong sense of community; group routines. These are like the heartbeats of our shared experiences, keeping us connected and supported.

What Exactly Are Group Routines?

Group routines are like those comforting traditions or activities that a bunch of folks in your community do together. They could be as simple as a weekly card game, a monthly potluck dinner, or more elaborate, like celebrating cultural festivals. The key is that they're shared and bring people closer.

Why Do Group Routines Matter?

Group routines play a crucial role in building a sense of togetherness and support in our communities: Hey there, let's talk about something that's as essential as air and water for humans - connecting with other people. It's the secret sauce that adds flavor and meaning to our lives, like a warm hug from a friend or a shared laugh with loved ones.

Human Connection is Vital: Just like we need food and water to survive, we need human connection for our emotional well-being. It's in our DNA to seek out social bonds. Connecting with people means you have a support system. Whether you're celebrating a success or facing a challenge, having someone by your side can make all the difference.

Think about your favorite memories. Chances are, they involve people you care about. Sharing experiences with others makes them more memorable and meaningful. Interacting with others exposes us to different ideas, perspectives, and cultures. It broadens our horizons and helps us grow as individuals.

Ways to Connect with People:

Active Listening: It's not just about talking; it's about truly listening to what others have to say. Show interest in their thoughts and feelings. Be present in the moment.

Authenticity: Be yourself. People appreciate genuineness. Pretending to be someone you're not won't lead to meaningful connections.

Shared Interests: Find common ground. Whether it's a hobby, a favorite book, or a passion for the outdoors, shared interests provide a great foundation for connection.

Quality Time: Spend time with people you care about. It could be a simple coffee date, a movie night, or a weekend getaway. Quality time builds strong bonds.

Empathy: Try to understand others' feelings and perspectives. Put yourself in their shoes. A little empathy goes a long way in building connections.

Communication: Clear and open communication is key. Express your thoughts and feelings honestly and encourage others to do the same.

Challenges and Solutions:

We often lead busy lives with work, family, and other commitments. But even small interactions, like a quick text or a phone call, can help maintain connections. Sometimes, we fear rejection or judgment. Remember that making connections involves some vulnerability. Not everyone will click, but those who do are worth it. In today's digital age, social media can sometimes feel overwhelming. Balance online interactions with real-world connections. Use technology to enhance, not replace, your relationships.

It can be challenging, but with effort and creativity, long-distance relationships can thrive. Schedule regular video calls, send surprise gifts, and plan visits when possible. Connecting with people is like tending to the garden of your life. It requires effort, care, and patience. But the beauty it adds to your world is immeasurable. So, reach out, listen, share, and embrace the connections that make your journey through life richer and more meaningful.

Creating a support network and building a strong sense of belonging. These elements are like the pillars that uphold our emotional well-being and enrich our lives. Just like a bundle of sticks is harder to break than a single twig, having a support network makes you more resilient. When you face challenges, whether big or small, having people to lean on can make all the difference.

Your support network can include family, friends, colleagues, or even support groups. Each provides a unique kind of support, from emotional comfort to practical advice. A support network is a two-way street. Just as you receive support, be open to giving it in return. It strengthens the bonds you share with others. Keep the lines of communication open. Share your thoughts and feelings with your support network and encourage them to do the same. Being there for one another fosters trust and understanding.

Building a Sense of Belonging:

Finding your "tribe" or community is like discovering a place where you fit in naturally. Seek out people who share your interests, values, or beliefs. Make an effort to include others. Extend a warm welcome to newcomers and make them feel like they belong. Inclusivity strengthens the bonds of your community.

Just like family traditions bring relatives together, creating community traditions fosters a sense of belonging. Whether it's a weekly gathering or an annual event, traditions help establish a shared identity. A sense of belonging thrives in an environment where individuals feel valued and accepted. Encourage empathy and kindness within your community.

Challenges and Solutions:

Finding Your Support Network: Sometimes, it can be challenging to find the right people to form your support network. Seek out local groups or online communities related to your interests or needs.

Overcoming Loneliness: Loneliness can hinder a sense of belonging. To combat this, make an effort to connect with others. Attend gatherings, join clubs, or volunteer for causes you care about.

Cultural and Social Differences: Differences in culture, background, or beliefs can sometimes create barriers to belonging. Embrace diversity and engage in open, respectful dialogue to bridge these gaps.

Maintaining Relationships: In our fast-paced world, it can be challenging to maintain relationships. Dedicate time to nurturing your connections, even in small ways, like sending a text or scheduling a regular catch-up.

Creating a support network and building a strong sense of belonging are like building a sturdy home for your emotional well-being. They provide shelter during life's storms and a warm hearth to return to. So, reach out to those who uplift you, and nurture the sense of belonging that makes you feel at home in the world.

Examples of Group Routines:

Let's take a peek at some everyday group routines:

Gathering friends or family for a game night is a fantastic routine. Whether it's board games, card games, or video games, it's a time for friendly competition and lots of laughter. Joining a community or charity group for volunteer activities can create a deep sense of purpose and camaraderie. Working together for a common cause strengthens bonds.

In the workplace, routines like celebrating birthdays, having weekly team meetings, or going for coffee breaks together foster teamwork and a sense of belonging among colleagues. Regular family dinners, where everyone sits down to share a meal and catch up on their day, are a cherished routine that strengthens family bonds.

Creating Your Own Group Routines

If you're keen on starting your own group routine in your community, here's how: Find something that your group of friends or community members is passionate about. It could be cooking, playing music, hiking, or any shared hobby.

Decide when you'll meet. It could be weekly, monthly, or even seasonally. Consistency is key to making it a part of everyone's routine. Infuse your routine with meaning. Whether it's sharing personal stories, contributing to a shared project, or simply enjoying each other's company, make it enjoyable and memorable.

As your routine becomes a regular part of your community's life, create traditions within it. It could be an annual theme party, a special ceremony, or a meaningful gesture that becomes your signature. Be open to people from different backgrounds and perspectives. Inclusivity enriches the experience and helps build a more diverse and vibrant community.

Engaging in group routines for community support is like tending to a garden of relationships. It's about nurturing connections, fostering a sense of belonging, and providing a safety net for one another. So, whether it's a weekly movie night, a monthly knitting circle, or an annual community clean-up day, embrace these routines as the threads that weave your community together.

Scott Anthony

Chapter 7

Beyond Physical Balance

Exploring the Connection Between Physical, Mental and Emotional Balance

Today, let's talk about something super important: finding that sweet balance between our bodies, minds, and emotions. You know, it's like making sure all the ingredients in your favorite recipe are just right to create a perfect dish. So, let's dive into it in a simple and easy way.

First off, physical balance. It's all about keeping our bodies healthy and in tip-top shape. This means eating good stuff like fruits and veggies, getting some exercise, and making sure we catch enough Z's at night. Remember, our bodies are like machines, and they need regular maintenance to keep running smoothly.

Now, let's talk about the mental side of things. Our brains are like a muscle, too. To keep them sharp, we can challenge ourselves with puzzles, learn new things, and even take some time to relax and de-stress. Just like you'd exercise your body, it's important to exercise your brain to stay mentally balanced.

Lastly, emotions. We all have them, right? Sometimes they're as unpredictable as the weather! But it's crucial to understand and manage our feelings. Talking to friends or family, practicing deep breathing, or even enjoying a hobby can help keep our emotions in check. Remember, it's perfectly normal to feel different emotions, but the key is not to let them overwhelm you.

Now, you might wonder why these three things are connected. Well, when we take care of our bodies, our minds and emotions benefit too. For example, when you get some exercise, your brain releases happy chemicals that can improve your mood. And when you're feeling good physically, it's easier to handle stress and emotions.

So, here's the bottom line, my friends: finding that balance between physical, mental, and emotional well-being is like the secret sauce to a happy and healthy life. It's not about being perfect or doing everything right all the time. It's about making small, manageable changes that work for you.

Take it one step at a time, enjoy the journey, and don't forget to savor all the delicious moments in life. After all, life is all about finding your balance and dancing to your own rhythm.

Strategies for Managing Stress, Anxiety and Mood

Let's talk about some simple and easy ways to deal with stress, anxiety, and mood swings.

Life can get a bit overwhelming at times, especially as we get older, but there are some tricks and tips that can make things a bit smoother. So, let's dive right in!

Stress, anxiety, and mood are interconnected aspects of mental and emotional well-being that can significantly impact a person's quality of life. Let's explore each of them individually:

Stress: Stress is a natural response to challenging or threatening situations. It can be both physical and psychological. When you perceive a situation as stressful, your body's "fight or flight" response is triggered, leading to physiological changes like increased heart rate, heightened alertness, and the release of stress hormones like cortisol. Short-term stress can be beneficial as it can help you respond to immediate threats, but chronic stress can have detrimental effects on your physical and mental health.

Anxiety: Anxiety is a natural and adaptive response to stressors, but it becomes problematic when it is excessive, irrational, or chronic. Generalized Anxiety Disorder (GAD) is a common anxiety disorder characterized by excessive and uncontrollable worry about everyday life events. Other anxiety disorders include panic disorder, social anxiety disorder, and specific phobias, each with its own set of symptoms and triggers.

Mood: Mood refers to a more generalized and sustained emotional state. It encompasses feelings like happiness, sadness, anger, and contentment. Mood disorders, such as major depressive disorder (depression) and bipolar disorder, are characterized by persistent disruptions in mood. Depression is characterized by persistent feelings of sadness, hopelessness, and a lack of interest or pleasure in activities.

Bipolar disorder involves extreme mood swings between depressive episodes and periods of mania or hypomania (elevated mood, energy, and activity levels).

Breathe Deeply: So, there I was, sitting in my favorite old armchair, feeling all knotted up with worry. Life can be a real rollercoaster, you know? But then I remembered something simple yet powerful: breathing.

Yep, it's as easy as it sounds. When those pesky stress and anxiety feelings start creeping in, just take a moment and think about your breath. Close your eyes if you want or keep them open - whatever feels right for you.

Start by taking a nice, deep breath in through your nose, like you're smelling a bouquet of fresh flowers. Count to four as you do it. One, two, three, four. Hold that breath for four beats, like you're savoring the aroma. And then, let it all out gently through your mouth, like you're blowing out a birthday candle. Another count of four.

It's like hitting a mini reset button for your mind. Your thoughts might be racing a hundred miles an hour, but this simple breathing exercise can slow them down. It's like a gentle wave washing over your worries.

I've found that doing this a few times whenever life gets a bit too crazy can make a big difference. It's a little moment of calm in the storm, a reminder that we have the power to soothe ourselves, no matter what's going on around us.

So, next time you're feeling a tad overwhelmed, just remember to breathe deeply. It's your secret weapon against stress, and it's always right there with you, ready to help you find your peace again.

Stay Active: Absolutely, staying active is a great way to keep your body and mind feeling good! You don't have to be a fitness guru or run a marathon to stay active. Just a little bit of movement can make a big difference in how you feel.

One simple way to stay active is by taking a leisurely stroll in the park. It's a lovely way to enjoy the outdoors, get some fresh air, and maybe even spot some birds or squirrels along the way. Plus, it's easy on your joints and doesn't require any fancy equipment.

If you're looking for something a bit more structured, you could try some gentle stretching exercises. Stretching can help improve your flexibility, reduce stiffness, and make everyday activities easier. You can find easy-to-follow stretching routines online or ask a friend to show you some simple moves.

Another fun option is joining a senior fitness class. These classes are designed with seniors in mind and are usually low-impact and friendly. You'll get to socialize with others while keeping your body active and healthy.

Remember, the goal is to move your body and have fun while doing it. So, whether it's a casual walk, gentle stretches, or a fitness class, find what works best for you and enjoy the benefits of staying active!

Talk it Out: Absolutely, talking it out can be a real game-changer, especially when you're going through tough times. Think of it like having a good old chat with a buddy over a cup of tea or coffee. Sharing your worries with a friend or family member can be like opening a pressure valve – it releases some of that built-up stress.

You don't need to worry about using fancy words or being super formal when you talk to someone you trust. Just be yourself and let it flow naturally. Sometimes, even the act of saying your worries out loud can help you see things from a different perspective.

So, next time you're feeling overwhelmed or just need to vent, don't hesitate to pick up the phone, meet for a chat, or even have a virtual video call. It's like a mini-therapy session that can do wonders for your mental well-being. Plus, you never know, your friend might have some great advice or a funny story to share that'll make you smile. Remember, you're not alone – there are people who care about you and are willing to listen.

Mindfulness and Meditation: Absolutely, you're on the right track! Mindfulness and meditation might sound a bit fancy, but trust me, it's simpler than you think. You don't need to be a Zen master or sit cross-legged for hours. Let's break it down:

Imagine you're sitting in a comfy chair, sipping a cup of tea, and enjoying the moment. That's mindfulness! It's about being fully present, right here, right now. No need to worry about the past or future.

Now, meditation. Think of it as a mini-vacation for your mind. You can do it for just a few minutes. Find a quiet spot, sit comfortably, and close your eyes if you want. Then, focus on something easy, like your breath going in and out. Inhale slowly, exhale gently. If your mind starts to wander (which happens to all of us!), simply bring it back to your breath.

Another trick is to use a calming word like "peace" or "relax" and repeat it quietly to yourself. It's like a mental reset button that helps calm your thoughts.

Meditation helps reduce stress and clear the mental clutter. It's like taking a break for your mind. So, don't stress about becoming a meditation pro. Just give it a try, and you might find it surprisingly relaxing and refreshing. Remember, it's all about simplicity and finding a little peace in the hustle and bustle of life.

You know, the beauty of mindfulness is that you can practice it anytime, anywhere. Whether you're enjoying a meal, taking a leisurely stroll, or even doing the dishes, you can be mindful. It's as simple as paying full attention to what you're doing in that very moment. So, next time you're savoring a slice of pie, savor it fully. Feel the texture, taste the flavors, and relish each bite. That's mindfulness in action – being fully engaged with the here and now.

Now, let's talk about some practical tips for meditation, especially for beginners. First, find a comfy spot where you won't be disturbed. It could be your favorite chair, a cozy corner, or even your bed. There are no strict rules here; comfort is key.

Next, set a timer for a short period, say 5 or 10 minutes, so you won't have to worry about checking the clock. Close your eyes if you'd like, but it's not mandatory. The important thing is to be comfortable.

As you focus on your breath or your calming word, you might notice that your mind starts to wander. That's completely normal – our minds are like playful puppies, always running around. When this happens, don't be hard on yourself. Just gently bring your attention back to your breath or your word. It's a bit like training that playful puppy; it takes practice, but it gets easier with time.

One more thing, meditation isn't about emptying your mind completely. It's more like creating a quiet space within your thoughts. You might still have thoughts popping in – that's okay. Acknowledge them and gently guide your focus back to your breath or your word.

With practice, you'll find that these short meditation sessions can do wonders for reducing stress and bringing a sense of calm into your life. It's like a little mental vacation that you can take whenever you need it. So, give it a shot, and remember, there's no need to rush or be perfect at it. It's all about simplicity, relaxation, and being kind to yourself. Enjoy your journey into mindfulness and meditation!

Hobbies and Interests: Hobbies and Interests: Discovering What Makes You Happy

Life is a journey and as we get older, it's important to find things that make us smile. One of the best ways to do that is by picking up a hobby or exploring your interests. It's like giving yourself a little gift of happiness.

Now, you might be wondering, "What kind of hobby should I take up?" Well, the good news is there are countless options, and you don't have to be an expert in anything. It's all about having fun and enjoying yourself. Let's dive into a few ideas:

1. **Gardening**: If you have a green thumb or just love being outdoors, gardening could be your thing. You don't need a big garden – a few pots on a balcony or a small indoor plant can work wonders. Watching your plants grow and bloom can be incredibly satisfying.

2. **Knitting or Crocheting**: These crafts are not only relaxing but also great for making beautiful gifts for your loved ones. You can knit scarves, blankets, or even cute baby clothes. Plus, it's an excellent way to keep your hands and mind engaged.

3. **Painting or Drawing**: You don't have to be the next Picasso to enjoy painting or sketching. Grab some brushes, paints, and paper, and let your creativity flow. Whether it's abstract art or a simple landscape, it's all about expressing yourself.

4. **Playing an Instrument**: Always dreamt of playing the guitar or the piano? Well, it's never too late to start. Learning an instrument can be a fulfilling journey. Plus, you'll be the life of the party when you bust out a tune at family gatherings!

The best thing about hobbies is that they take your mind off everyday worries. When you're engrossed in your favorite activity, time seems to fly, and you'll find yourself feeling happier and more relaxed.

So, go ahead and explore what piques your interest. Maybe it's something on this list, or maybe it's something entirely different, like birdwatching, cooking, or even writing your memoirs. The key is to have fun and enjoy every moment of it.

Remember, there's no rush, no pressure, and no need to be perfect. It's all about finding joy in the little things. Happy hobby hunting, and here's to a happier, more fulfilling life!

Healthy Eating: Absolutely, let's dive deeper into the wonderful world of healthy eating; in a way that's easy to understand and follow for everyone, especially seniors!

Picture your body as a car. Just like a car needs good fuel to run smoothly, your body needs the right kind of food to stay healthy and happy. So, what's the secret recipe for a happy body and mind?

1. Fruits and Veggies: These colorful treasures are like nature's vitamins. They're packed with nutrients that can boost your energy, make your skin glow, and keep your digestion in check. Plus, they're delicious! Try to have a variety of them on your plate – from apples to zucchinis.

2. Whole Grains: Think of whole grains like your body's best friend. They give you long-lasting energy and help you feel full and satisfied. Choose whole grain bread, pasta, and rice over the white stuff for extra benefits.

3. Drink Up: Water is like magic potion for your body. It keeps your joints moving smoothly, your skin hydrated, and your brain sharp. Sip on water throughout the day to stay refreshed. Tea and unsweetened coffee count too!

4. Proteins: These are the building blocks for your muscles and tissues. Lean meats, poultry, fish, eggs, and beans are great sources of protein. They'll help you stay strong and energetic.

5. Healthy Fats: Not all fats are bad. In fact, your body needs some healthy fats for a well-oiled machine. Olive oil, avocados, nuts, and seeds are your friends in this department. They're good for your heart and brain.

Now, you might be thinking, "What about treats?" Well, there's room for those too! It's all about balance. Treat yourself to your favorite dessert or snack once in a while. Just remember, moderation is the key.

Remember, eating well isn't about following complicated rules. It's about choosing real, whole foods that make you feel good. When you nourish your body with these goodies, you'll have more energy to do the things you love, and you'll likely feel happier too!

So, go ahead, fill your plate with colorful veggies, savor the taste of fresh fruits, and don't forget to raise a glass of water to your health. Here's to a happy and healthy you!

Limit News and Social Media: Absolutely, folks! Let's chat about a simple way to take care of your mental well-being: limiting your time on the news and social media.

You know, in today's world, it's super tempting to scroll through Facebook, Twitter, or watch the news all day long. But here's the thing – too much of that stuff, especially when it's all about bad news, can really bring your mood down.

So, what can we do? Well, it's as easy as setting some boundaries. Maybe try to limit your screen time. You don't have to be glued to your phone or computer all day. Take a break, go for a walk, or just do something you enjoy. Trust me, a little break from all the news and updates can make you feel so much better.

Remember, it's all about finding a balance. Stay informed, but don't let the constant stream of information overwhelm you. Your mental well-being is important, so take those breaks and enjoy the simple things in life!

Get Enough Rest: Getting a good night's sleep is like giving your body a superpower boost! It's not just about feeling less tired; it's about helping your body and mind stay in tip-top shape.

So, let's talk about why sleep is so important. First off, it's like a magic potion for your well-being. Imagine a potion that could make you feel happier, more alert, and less stressed. Well, that's what sleep does for you!

Here's the scoop: when you get enough rest, your body gets a chance to recharge and repair itself. It's like a little army of repair workers going to town, fixing up any wear and tear from the day. Your brain also gets a chance to sort through all the things you learned and experienced, making sure everything is stored away neatly.

To make the most of this magical potion, try to stick to a regular sleep schedule. Going to bed and waking up at the same times every day can really help your body get into a groove. It's like telling your body, "Hey, it's time to rest now." And when you create a comfy bedtime routine, it's like adding an extra sprinkle of magic to your sleep. Maybe you like to read a book, have a warm cup of tea, or take a relaxing bath before bed – these little routines can signal to your body that it's time to wind down.

When you're well-rested, you're like a superhero. You can handle stress better, think more clearly, and even stay in a better mood. So, don't underestimate the power of a good night's sleep. It's your secret weapon for feeling your best and taking on each day with a smile!

Laugh It Out: Laughter is like a magical elixir that can instantly brighten up your day. It's one of those simple pleasures in life that can work wonders for your overall well-being.

Think about it; how great does it feel when you burst into laughter, your belly shaking, tears of joy streaming down your cheeks? It's like a mini vacation from all your worries and stress. And guess what? It's completely free!

So, what can you do to bring more laughter into your life? Well, there are plenty of options, and you can choose whatever tickles your funny bone.

One classic way to get a good laugh is by watching a funny movie or TV show. Pick a comedy that you love, or maybe explore a new one. Sometimes, all it takes is a hilarious character or a clever punchline to get you giggling.

If you prefer a quieter approach, you can dive into a joke book or simply search for jokes online. There's a treasure trove of humor out there, from classic knock-knock jokes to witty one-liners. Share them with friends or family, and you'll find yourself in fits of laughter in no time.

And speaking of friends and family, spending time with people who make you laugh is another surefire way to brighten your day. It could be your grandkids telling their goofy stories, your best friend recounting their latest misadventures, or even just chatting with a neighbor who has a knack for humor.

Remember, laughter isn't just about amusement; it has genuine health benefits too. It can reduce stress, boost your mood, and even strengthen your immune system. Plus, it's contagious; when you laugh, those around you are likely to catch the laughter bug too.

So, don't underestimate the power of laughter. It's a natural mood booster and an instant remedy for those moments when life feels a bit heavy. Keep those funny movies, joke books, and hilarious friends close by, and let the laughter flow. After all, a hearty laugh is one of life's simplest and greatest pleasures!

Seek Professional Help: Let's talk about something important: getting a little help when life throws some tough stuff your way. It's like having a trusty umbrella for a rainy day; sometimes, we all need a bit of extra support.

So, here's the deal: when life starts feeling like an uphill battle, it's totally okay to ask for a helping hand. And guess what? There are some fantastic folks out there called therapists or counselors who are experts at helping you sort through the tough stuff.

Now, I know what you might be thinking, "Do I really need to talk to a therapist? Is it a big deal?" Well, let me assure you, there's absolutely no shame in reaching out for a little professional support. We all go through rough patches, and these trained pros are there to lend an ear and offer some guidance.

Think of it this way: just like you'd visit a doctor when you're feeling under the weather, a therapist is like your emotional health doctor. They're really good at listening, understanding what's bothering you, and giving you tools to help you feel better.

Maybe you're dealing with the loss of a loved one, feeling overwhelmed with stress, or having trouble sleeping – therapists can help with all of that and more. They won't judge you, and they're bound by confidentiality, so what you share stays between you and them.

So, if you ever find yourself in a place where things are getting a bit too tough to handle solo, remember that there's a whole bunch of caring professionals out there just waiting to help you navigate life's challenges. It's a sign of strength, not weakness, to seek a little extra support when you need it.

Bottom line: don't hesitate to reach out to a therapist or counselor if you need it. They're like the friendly neighbors next door who always have a comforting cup of tea ready for you. So, take care of yourself and remember, it's okay to seek professional help when life gets a little too heavy. You've got this!

Remember, it's okay to have ups and downs; that's just part of life. These simple strategies can make the journey a bit smoother, and it's all about finding what works best for you. So take a deep breath, smile, and take one step at a time. You've got this!

Cultivating Gratitude and Mindfulness in Daily Life

We're going to chat about something super important but also wonderfully simple – cultivating gratitude and mindfulness in our daily lives. Now, you might be thinking, "What's all the fuss about?" Well, let's dive in and find out!

Gratitude, in a nutshell, is all about appreciating the good stuff in our lives, big or small. It's like saying "thank you" to the universe for the simple joys, like a warm cup of tea on a chilly morning or a smile from a friend. It's about focusing on what we have, rather than what we lack.

Mindfulness, on the other hand, is about being present in the moment. It's taking a break from the constant hustle and bustle to savor life's little details – the scent of fresh flowers, the taste of a delicious meal, or the feeling of the sun on your skin. It's like hitting the pause button and really soaking in the beauty around you.

So, how can we bring more gratitude and mindfulness into our everyday lives, especially as seniors? Well, it's easier than you might think!

Morning Gratitude Routine: Start your day with a simple gratitude routine. Maybe keep a journal by your bedside and jot down three things you're thankful for each morning. It could be the chirping of birds outside your window, the cozy blanket that keeps you warm, or the memories of days gone by.

Mindful Meals: Let's chat about something we all do every day – eating. We all know that mealtime can sometimes feel like a race, especially with our busy lives. But have you ever thought about slowing down a bit and truly enjoying your food? That's what we call "mindful eating," and it's not as complicated as it sounds.

So, picture this: you're sitting at the table, ready to dig into your meal. The first thing you might want to do is put away those distractions. Yep, that means no TV, no scrolling through your smartphone, and definitely no work emails. It's time to focus on the deliciousness right in front of you.

Now, take a moment to look at your plate. Notice the vibrant colors – maybe there's a rainbow of veggies, or the warm, inviting hue of your favorite comfort food. Pay attention to the textures; is it crispy, creamy, or tender? And when you take that first bite, really savor it. Feel the flavors dance on your taste buds. Is it sweet, salty, or maybe a little spicy?

You see, when we slow down and pay attention to our food, something magical happens. We start to appreciate the simple act of nourishing our bodies. It's not just about filling up; it's about enjoying every mouthful, connecting with the flavors, and taking a break from the hustle and bustle of life.

So, the next time you sit down for a meal, give this mindful eating thing a try. Put away those distractions, savor each bite, and let your senses guide you. You'll be surprised at how much more you can enjoy your food and the moment. Happy eating, my friends!

Nature Strolls: If you can, take a leisurely walk in the park or your garden. Notice the beauty of the flowers, the rustling leaves, and the gentle breeze. It's like a mini-escape to a natural wonderland.

Gratitude for Friends and Family: Reach out to loved ones and express your gratitude for their presence in your life. A simple "thank you" or a heartfelt message can go a long way in strengthening your bonds.

Breathing Breaks: Sometimes, all you need is a few deep breaths to center yourself. Take a moment to inhale slowly, feel the air fill your lungs, and then exhale. It's a quick way to bring mindfulness into your day, no matter where you are.

Bedtime Reflection: Before you drift off to sleep, reflect on the positive moments of your day. Even if it was a tough day, find something small to be grateful for. It sets the tone for peaceful sleep and a fresh start tomorrow.

Technology Timeout: Take short breaks from technology. We all love our gadgets, but sometimes they can whisk us away from the present moment. Try turning off your phone or computer for a little while and just be with yourself or enjoy a good book.

Unplug at Meals: When you sit down to enjoy a meal, put away the screens and engage with your dining companions. Sharing stories and laughter over a meal can be a beautiful way to connect and savor the moment.

Enjoy a Hobby: Do you have a hobby you adore? Whether it's knitting, gardening, painting, or playing an instrument, immersing yourself in an activity you love can be incredibly mindful. It's like a mini-vacation for your mind.

Practice Gratefulness in Tough Times: Life has its ups and downs, and that's okay. Even during challenging moments, try to find a silver lining. Perhaps it's a lesson learned or the strength you didn't know you had. This practice can help you navigate rough waters with grace.

Simplify Your Space: Consider decluttering your living space. A tidy, organized home can bring a sense of calm and mindfulness. Plus, you might uncover forgotten treasures that make you smile.

Connect with Nature: If possible, spend time outdoors. Even a few minutes in your garden or on your balcony can help you feel more connected to the natural world. Listen to the birds, feel the earth beneath your feet, and breathe in the fresh air.

Share Gratitude Stories: When you get together with friends or family, ask each person to share something they're grateful for. It's a heartwarming way to strengthen bonds and inspire one another.

Smile and Laugh: Don't forget to smile and laugh. They say laughter is the best medicine, and it's true! Whether it's a funny movie, a joke, or a silly memory, a good laugh can instantly lift your spirits.

Learn to Say No: Sometimes, practicing mindfulness means respecting your own boundaries. It's okay to say no to commitments that overwhelm you. This helps you focus on what truly matters.

Remember, there's no right or wrong way to embrace gratitude and mindfulness. It's about finding what works best for you and adding a sprinkle of mindfulness to your day. You've got this, and every small step you take brings you closer to a more mindful and grateful life.

So, keep it simple, keep it real, and keep embracing the beauty of each moment. Life is a gift, and practicing gratitude and mindfulness helps us cherish it all the more. Here's to a life filled with gratitude, mindfulness, and the simple joys that make it all worthwhile!

Testimonials from Seniors Who Have Benefited from the Routines

Sure, I'd be happy to help you create some casual and simple content based on testimonials from seniors who have benefited from routines. Here are a few testimonials in a relaxed and straightforward style:

Betty, 72: "I used to feel a bit lost after retirement, but then I started incorporating some daily routines into my life. It's amazing how something as simple as a morning walk and a cup of tea can bring so much joy. These little routines have given me a sense of purpose and a routine that I cherish." Betty, 72, knows the secret to a happy retirement – daily routines! You might think retirement means endless free time, but it can sometimes leave you feeling a bit lost. Betty felt the same way, but she discovered that adding a few simple routines to her life made a world of difference.

One of Betty's favorite routines is taking a leisurely morning walk. It doesn't have to be a marathon, just a gentle stroll to wake up her body and mind. The fresh air and the sounds of nature are like a soothing balm for her soul. It's a great way to start the day feeling refreshed and energized.

And what's a morning walk without a cup of tea, right? Betty swears by her daily cuppa. It's not just about the tea itself; it's the whole experience. She brews her favorite tea, finds a cozy spot to sit, and takes her time sipping it. It's a moment of calm and relaxation, a time to reflect and enjoy the little things in life.

These simple routines might not seem like much, but they've given Betty a sense of purpose and a routine that she absolutely cherishes. They've become anchors in her day, something to look forward to, and a source of joy. Plus, they're easy to incorporate into her life, making every day a little brighter.

So, whether you're retired or not, take a page out of Betty's book and consider adding some simple daily routines to your routine. It might just be the key to finding more happiness and contentment in your life. After all, it's the little things that often matter the most.

George, 78: Meet George, who's 78 years young! George's grandkids did something pretty cool – they got him into meditation. Now, you might be thinking, "Meditation? Isn't that for monks and yoga gurus?" Well, not exactly! George here will tell you how it's changed his life in the simplest and most chill way.

So, George wasn't too sure about this meditation stuff at first. Like, who could blame him? But guess what? He gave it a shot! And now? He's loving it.

He says it's like a "mental spa." Imagine that! Just like how you go to a spa to relax your body, meditation does that for your mind. It's like a mini-vacation for your brain – no luggage required!

George says it keeps him calm and focused. And who wouldn't want that, right? Life can be a bit crazy sometimes, but with meditation, you've got a secret weapon to stay cool and collected.

And here's the best part: George wants you to know that it's NEVER too late to try new things! Whether you're 18 or 80, you can dive into something new and exciting. Meditation is just one of those things that can make life a whole lot better.

So, if you've been thinking about trying meditation, why not give it a whirl? You might discover your own "mental spa" and find that inner calm and focus that George did. Who knows? It could be your next favorite thing!

Remember, life is an adventure, and George is living proof that there's always room for something new, no matter your age. So go on, give meditation a try, and who knows, you might just surprise yourself!

Martha, 68: "Cooking used to be a chore, but now it's a delightful routine for me. I've started experimenting with new recipes, and every evening, I whip up something special. It's brought a new flavor to my life, quite literally!" Meet Martha, a vibrant 68-year-old who's discovered the joy of cooking later in life. For her, cooking isn't a dull chore anymore; it's become a delightful daily routine. She's taken up the spatula and apron to whip up new and exciting recipes that add a tasty twist to her evenings.

You see, Martha's found that cooking isn't just about food; it's about flavoring life itself. She's gone from the usual dinner routine to a culinary adventure every evening. No fancy chef's hat or high-tech gadgets needed – just a pinch of curiosity and a dash of enthusiasm.

Martha's secret? She's not afraid to try something new. Whether it's a spicy Thai curry, a comforting bowl of homemade soup, or a batch of freshly baked chocolate chip cookies, Martha's kitchen is always buzzing with delicious experiments. And guess what? You can do it too!

Imagine the satisfaction of creating a mouthwatering meal from scratch, the smell of herbs and spices filling your kitchen, and the taste of a perfectly seasoned dish on your plate. It's like a little party for your taste buds every day.

So, if you're a senior looking to add some zest to your life, consider following in Martha's footsteps. You don't need to be a gourmet chef or have a fancy kitchen – all you need is the willingness to explore and the joy of savoring every bite.

Cooking can be your delightful daily routine too. Who knows what new flavors and adventures you'll discover in your own kitchen? So, grab that recipe book, put on your favorite music, and let's get cooking!

Sam, 75: That's awesome to hear! Reading a chapter of a book every night sounds like a great way to unwind and keep your mind active. It's like a little adventure right before bedtime, isn't it?

I totally get what you mean. Sometimes, life gets so busy, and we forget to make time for ourselves. But reading is a wonderful way to escape into different worlds, meet new characters, and go on exciting journeys—all from the comfort of your favorite chair.

You know, it's never too late to start reading more. And it doesn't have to be a big, fancy novel. You can pick up any book that interests you, whether it's a thrilling mystery, a heartwarming romance, or even some funny jokes in a joke book. The best part is, you're in control of your adventure, and you can explore at your own pace.

Plus, reading has a sneaky way of expanding our horizons. You can learn about new cultures, history, and so much more, all while enjoying a good story. It's like having a world of knowledge at your fingertips.

So, keep up the great work! Your nightly reading routine is a fantastic way to add a little extra excitement to your day and keep your mind sharp. Who knows where your next adventure between the pages will take you? Happy reading!

Eleanor, 70: Eleanor, you've hit the nail on the head! Gardening is like a daily dose of calmness and joy, no matter your age.

I mean, who needs a fancy spa day when you've got your own little green haven right in your backyard or even on your windowsill? Watching those plants grow is like witnessing a miracle every day.

I'll tell you, I've seen my fair share of stressful days, but there's something about being surrounded by nature that just melts it all away. The gentle rustle of leaves, the chirping of birds, and the scent of blooming flowers – it's pure magic for the soul.

So, to all the seniors out there, if you haven't already, give gardening a try! You don't need a green thumb or fancy tools. Just a little bit of soil, some seeds or small plants, and a whole lot of love. It's a wonderful way to connect with nature, stay active, and find your daily dose of tranquility, just like Eleanor.

When your flowers bloom or you harvest your first homegrown tomato, the sense of accomplishment is priceless. So go on, grab a shovel, get your hands dirty, and let Mother Nature work her wonders on you. Your little garden paradise is waiting! "Gardening has become my daily therapy. Tending to my plants, watching them grow, and being surrounded by nature is like a daily dose of tranquility. It's amazing how a small garden can bring so much peace."

John, 73: That's great to hear, John! I remember when you first mentioned trying Tai Chi a few months ago. It's wonderful that you've found something you enjoy so much and that it's making such a positive difference in your life.

I bet it's been quite the journey. Can you share a bit more about how you got into Tai Chi and what your experience has been like?

John chuckled, "Sure thing! Well, you know, I was feeling a bit stiff and unsteady on my feet. My grandkids would always invite me to play in the park, and I'd worry about falling or not being able to keep up. That's when my neighbor, Sarah, suggested I try Tai Chi. She's been practicing it for years and said it's like a gentle exercise that's perfect for seniors like us."

He continued, "So, I thought, why not give it a shot? I found a local Tai Chi class at the community center. On the first day, I was a bit nervous, not knowing what to expect. But as soon as I stepped into the room, I felt this calm and welcoming atmosphere. There were people of all ages, and the instructor, Mr. Chang, had this soothing presence that put me at ease."

John's eyes sparkled with enthusiasm as he continued, "We started with some simple warm-up exercises and then gradually moved into the Tai Chi forms. Mr. Chang explained that Tai Chi is like a slow, flowing dance inspired by nature. I could immediately feel the grace and beauty in the movements. It wasn't about pushing my limits; it was about moving with the rhythm of my own body and breath."

He took a deep breath, savoring the memories, "Over the weeks, I started noticing changes. My balance improved, and I felt more stable on my feet. I no longer worried about falling when I played with my grandkids. Even my doctor noticed my blood pressure was better. But you know what the best part is? It's the sense of peace and mindfulness that Tai Chi brings. It's like a mini vacation for my mind every time I practice."

I asked John if he had any advice for others thinking about trying Tai Chi, and he grinned, "Oh, absolutely! I'd say don't be shy. Give it a try. It's not about being super flexible or fit; it's about connecting with your body and finding harmony within. Plus, it's a fantastic way to meet new friends. I've made some wonderful companions in my Tai Chi class, and we often go out for tea after our sessions."

As we wrapped up our chat, John left me with a heartfelt thought, "Tai Chi has added a whole new chapter to my life. It's never too late to start something new and feel healthier and more energetic. If I can do it at 73, anyone can!"

Ruth, 80: Ruth, 80, leaned back in her cozy armchair, a contented smile on her face as she reminisced about her family's Sunday potluck dinners. She had been hosting these gatherings for as long as she could remember, and they were truly the highlight of her week.

"You know, dear," she began, her eyes twinkling with fond memories, "our Sunday potlucks have been a tradition in our family for generations. It's a simple but heartwarming routine that keeps us all connected."

Ruth's family, a diverse bunch of generations, would gather at her home each Sunday evening, bringing with them dishes of all shapes and flavors. Her granddaughter, Sarah, would often whip up her famous mac 'n' cheese, and Ruth's son, Robert, never failed to bring a platter of mouthwatering barbeque ribs.

"We don't care about fancy recipes or gourmet cooking," Ruth explained with a chuckle. "What matters most is that we come together and share a meal made with love. That's what makes our Sunday dinners so special."

The dining table would be adorned with mismatched dishes and colorful tablecloths, adding a charming, homey touch to the gathering. As the family sat around, plates piled high with food, the room would be filled with the comforting aroma of various dishes mingling together.

"Stories, laughter, and love – that's what our Sunday dinners are all about," Ruth continued. "We'd share stories from the past, tales of our adventures, and even some embarrassing moments from our younger days. And you wouldn't believe the laughter that fills the room. It's like medicine for the soul."

Ruth's eyes sparkled as she remembered the times when her great-grandchildren would bring along their drawings and tell stories of their school adventures. "They keep us young at heart," she said with a grin. "Their innocence and enthusiasm remind us of the simple joys in life."

As the years went by, some things changed. The hairstyles, the fashion, and even the recipes evolved. Yet, one thing remained constant – the love and togetherness shared at their Sunday potluck dinners.

"Nowadays," Ruth mused, "our gatherings are a bit smaller, but the love is as big as ever. We might use a bit more salt than we used to, and some of us need a little help getting up from the table, but our hearts are still young and full of joy."

And so, every Sunday, Ruth and her family continued their cherished tradition, a simple yet powerful reminder of the importance of staying connected, sharing stories, and savoring the moments of togetherness. For Ruth, it was a tradition that filled her heart with warmth and made her grateful for the simple joys of life.

Frank, 76: Frank, 76, sat in his cozy little art studio, surrounded by canvases and paintbrushes. He chuckled to himself, thinking about how he had stumbled upon this newfound hobby of painting during his retirement years.

"You know," Frank began, "I never thought I'd be the type to pick up a paintbrush. But there's something magical about it. It's like a whole new world opens up when I dip that brush into the paint."

Frank's eyes sparkled with excitement as he continued, "I'm no Picasso, that's for sure. But it doesn't matter. What matters is how it makes me feel. It's therapeutic, you know? When I have a canvas and some colors in front of me, I forget about all my worries. It's a wonderful escape from the everyday."

He picked up a brush and started to blend some soft blues and pinks together on his current canvas. "I've painted landscapes, flowers, even a portrait of my old dog, Max," Frank said with a grin. "Every stroke of the brush, every dab of color, it's like I'm adding a piece of myself to the world. It's a form of self-expression I never knew I had in me."

As he painted, Frank's hands moved with a graceful rhythm, and he seemed completely at ease. "Some days," he said, "I lose track of time in here. My wife, Mary, has to remind me to come out for dinner. But I don't mind. It's worth it."

He paused for a moment, looking at the canvas, which was beginning to take shape as a serene seascape. "You see," Frank concluded, "retirement isn't just about slowing down; it's about finding new ways to enjoy life. And for me, painting has become one of the most beautiful and fulfilling parts of my retirement journey."

Alice, 71: Alice, 71, continued to brighten her days by dedicating her time to the local animal shelter. Every week, without fail, she'd stroll through the shelter's doors with a warm smile on her face. The moment she stepped inside, she was greeted by a chorus of barks, meows, and wagging tails that made her heart swell.

Alice had always loved animals, and her retirement had given her the perfect opportunity to nurture that passion. She didn't have her own pets anymore, but the shelter was like her extended family. She'd grown close to the shelter staff, who appreciated her dedication and kindness.

Her routine was simple but meaningful. Alice would spend her mornings helping to clean the kennels and cages, making sure each furry resident had a clean and cozy space. She'd chat with the shelter workers and share stories about her own pets from years past. It was a bit like a therapy session, both for her and the animals.

After the cleaning was done, Alice's favorite part of the day began. She'd walk through the aisles, offering pets and pats to all the animals. Each one had a unique personality, and Alice could tell you all about them. There was Max, the energetic Labrador who never seemed to run out of enthusiasm, and Lucy, the shy tabby cat who had finally started to trust humans again, thanks to Alice's gentle approach.

As she sat on the floor, surrounded by furry friends, Alice felt a deep sense of purpose. She knew that her presence brought comfort and happiness to these animals, many of whom had been through tough times. And in return, they filled her life with joy and companionship.

Alice often encouraged her fellow seniors to join her at the shelter. She'd tell them, "It's like having a bunch of grandpets without the responsibility!" Her friends would chuckle and nod, some of them eventually taking her up on the offer.

Volunteering at the animal shelter wasn't just a routine of compassion for Alice; it was a lifeline, a way to stay connected to the world and give back in her own special way. And as long as she had the strength to do it, she knew she'd keep coming back, week after week, to share her love and care with those furry friends who needed it most.

Bob, 69:   Bob, 69, chuckled as he settled into his favorite porch chair, the early morning sun warming his face. The scent of freshly brewed coffee wafted from the mug cradled in his hands, and he took a slow sip, savoring the comforting warmth.

Every day, rain or shine, Bob started his morning just like this. His porch, with its creaky old wooden floor and a comfy chair that had seen better days, was his sanctuary. He leaned back, eyes half-closed, and let the soothing symphony of chirping birds and distant laughter serenade him.

As he watched the world awaken, Bob couldn't help but smile. The bustling neighborhood seemed to come to life right before his eyes. Kids with backpacks ran down the sidewalk, their laughter filling the air, while the early risers jogged by, exchanging friendly waves. A mail carrier on his trusty bike rolled up, delivering letters and packages with a friendly nod.

Bob's eyes drifted to the trees lining the street, their leaves swaying gently in the breeze. They whispered stories of seasons past and secrets shared by young lovers. His porch, too, held its own tales of countless mornings spent in quiet contemplation.

He took another sip of coffee, feeling the rich, dark brew warm his soul. His wrinkled hands curled around the mug, a symbol of comfort in a rapidly changing world. The aroma of coffee mingled with the fragrance of blooming flowers in his garden, a small patch of colorful paradise that brought joy to his heart.

It was in these moments, as the world hurried by, that Bob found solace. He didn't need fancy gadgets or elaborate plans. No, his daily routine was a testament to the beauty of simplicity. It was a time to reflect on his life, to remember all the adventures he'd had and all the lessons he'd learned.

Bob gazed at the clear blue sky, grateful for the simple pleasures life offered. The chatter of neighbors passing by, the soft rustling of leaves, and the taste of that first morning coffee; it was all he needed. Each day was a gift, and he cherished it, one sip at a time.

As the sun climbed higher, casting long shadows across the porch, Bob continued to sit, content in the knowledge that the world would keep turning, and he would be right there, watching it go by, with a grateful heart and a cup of coffee in hand.

These testimonials show how seniors can find fulfillment and happiness through various routines, whether it's meditation, gardening, cooking, or simply enjoying a cup of coffee on the porch. It's all

Chapter 8

Sustaining a Lifetime of Balance

Tips for Maintaining a Lifelong Commitment to Balance Routines

Fellow life enthusiasts! Today, we're spicing things up and dishing out some seriously fun tips for keeping your life in perfect harmony. No fancy jargon or complicated theories here are just simple, everyday tricks to keep the good vibes flowing!

★ **Dance Through Life:** Life's a party, so why not dance your way through it? Put on your favorite tunes and have a dance-off in your living room. It's a great way to stay active and boost your mood at the same time!

★ **Treat Yourself... Gently:** We all love treats, right? Instead of overloading on that tub of ice cream, try some healthier alternatives. How about a delicious fruit smoothie or a colorful salad that's almost too pretty to eat?

★ **Embrace the Joy of Play**: Kids have all the fun with their games, but who says we can't join in? Board games, puzzles, or even a game of hide-and-seek with the grandkids – they all bring out the inner child in us.

★ **Nature Time:** Take a leisurely stroll in the park or your garden. Listen to the birds chirping, feel the sunshine on your face, and breathe in the fresh air. Mother Nature is the ultimate stress-buster.

★ **Hug It Out:** Hugs are magical. They release happy hormones and make you feel warm and fuzzy inside. Give your loved ones a big bear hug or even a hug to yourself. It's like a happiness injection!

★ **The Great Declutter Challenge:** Turn decluttering into a game. Set a timer and see how quickly you can tidy up a room. It's like a mini-Olympics for your home, and the prize is a neat and tidy space.

★ **Yoga for the Win:** Yoga isn't just for the super flexible. There are gentle yoga routines designed for everyone. Stretch those limbs, find your inner Zen, and strike a pose – it's like a yoga party for one!

★ **Learn While You Laugh:** Why not pick up a fun, quirky hobby? How about learning to juggle, do magic tricks, or master the art of making balloon animals? It's a surefire way to keep life interesting!

★ **Laugh Like There's No Tomorrow:** Laughter truly is the best medicine. Watch a comedy show, share funny stories with friends, or even indulge in some goofy, silly jokes. Let those belly laughs flow!

★ **Toast to Small Victories:** Every day is filled with little victories. Did you find your keys this morning? Hooray! Did you bake a batch of perfect cookies? Cheers! Celebrate these wins with a little dance or a tasty treat.

Remember, life is like a rollercoaster – full of ups and downs. But with these fun and fabulous tips, you'll be cruising through the twists and turns like a pro. So, go ahead, embrace the joy, dance like nobody's watching, and keep that smile shining bright. Life's too short not to have a blast!

Adapting Routines to Changing Needs and Abilities

Today, let's talk about something we all go through as we get older: changing needs and abilities. It's a part of life, and it's important to adapt our daily routines to match where we're at. No need to get all fancy or complicated – let's keep it simple and easy to understand.

- ❖ **Morning Routines:** Start your day right! If bending down to tie your shoes has become a bit tricky, consider slip-on shoes or Velcro closures. And if you love your morning cup of coffee but your hands shake a bit, a spill-proof mug might be a good friend.

- ❖ **Getting Dressed:** Buttons and zippers can be a hassle. Swap them out for clothes with elastic waistbands and pull-over tops. Dressing should be easy and stress-free.

- ❖ **Mealtime:** Cooking can be a joy, but if it's becoming a challenge, try pre-cut veggies or frozen meals that you can just pop in the microwave. There are also meal delivery services that bring tasty, balanced meals right to your door.

- ❖ **Technology**: Staying connected with loved ones is important, but technology can be confusing. Consider a smartphone with larger buttons or a tablet with simple apps for chatting and browsing.

- ❖ **Home Safety:** Falling can be a big concern. Make sure your home has good lighting, handrails in the right places, and non-slip mats. These small changes can make a big difference.

- ❖ **Exercise:** Staying active is vital, but you don't need to run marathons. Gentle exercises like walking, yoga, or tai chi can help keep you strong and balanced.

- ❖ **Medications:** If keeping track of your meds feels overwhelming, ask your doctor about pill organizers or automatic dispensers. They'll help you stay on top of your health.

❖ **Social Life:** Friends and family are important. If going out is tough, invite them over for a cozy gathering at home. You can still enjoy good company without the fuss.

❖ **Transportation:** If driving isn't an option anymore, look into public transportation, rideshares, or senior transportation services. Getting around should be convenient and stress-free.

❖ **Hobbies and Interests:** Pursue what you love! If gardening or crafts are getting harder, find ways to adapt – like raised garden beds or tools designed for easier use.

Remember, adapting your routines doesn't mean giving up the things you enjoy. It's about finding new ways to make life simpler and more enjoyable. Ask for help when you need it, and don't be afraid to explore new solutions. Your well-being is what matters most!

So, embrace the changes, keep it simple, and live life to the fullest!

Encouraging Family and Community Involvement

Encouraging family and community involvement is a wonderful way to stay connected, have fun, and make a positive impact in our lives. Whether you're a senior looking to get more involved, or you have a senior in your life who could use some encouragement, here are some easy and casual ideas to make it happen:

❖ **Family Game Nights:** Gather your family or friends for a fun game night. Whether it's card games, board games, or even a simple game of charades, it's a fantastic way to bond and share some laughs.

❖ **Community Potlucks:** Join a local community group or church that hosts potluck dinners. You can bring a dish to share and enjoy a meal with neighbors and friends. It's a great way to meet new people and strengthen existing connections.

❖ **Gardening Clubs:** If you have a green thumb or are interested in learning, consider joining a gardening club. Gardening not only connects you with nature but also with fellow gardening enthusiasts in your community.

❖ **Volunteer Opportunities:** Many organizations are always on the lookout for volunteers of all ages. Whether it's at a local library, animal shelter, or food bank, giving your time to help others is incredibly rewarding.

❖ **Attend Senior Centers:** Senior centers often host a variety of activities like exercise classes, arts and crafts, and social gatherings. It's a great place to meet new friends and stay active.

❖ **Neighborhood Walks:** Organize or join regular walks in your neighborhood. It's a simple way to get some exercise, enjoy the fresh air, and chat with neighbors along the way.

❖ **Share Your Skills:** Do you have a talent or skill you'd like to share? Whether it's cooking, knitting, or even telling stories, consider offering a workshop or class to your community. You'll be amazed at how much people appreciate your expertise.

❖ **Join a Book Club:** If you love to read, joining a book club is a fantastic way to connect with others who share your passion for books. Plus, it gives you the opportunity to discuss and debate your favorite stories.

❖ **Tech Help:** If you're a tech-savvy senior, consider offering your help to other seniors who might need assistance with their smartphones, tablets, or computers. It's a great way to bridge the generation gap.

❖ **Family Celebrations:** Don't forget to celebrate special occasions with your family. Birthdays, holidays, and anniversaries are perfect opportunities to come together, share meals, and create lasting memories.

Family and community involvement is about building connections and enjoying the company of others. It doesn't have to be formal or complicated. So, go ahead and take the first step; reach out to a neighbor, family member, or local group, and start enjoying the benefits of being involved in your community.

Resources for Further Exploration and Practice

You've learned some cool stuff, and now it's time to explore and practice more. Don't worry; we're keeping it super simple and easy-peasy! Let's take a look at a few additional ways to infuse your daily life with gratitude and mindfulness that feel like a walk in the park.

- **Ask a Friend or Family Member:** One of the best ways to learn is by chatting with someone you trust. Ask a friend or a family member if they know more about what you're interested in. Sometimes, they might even have some old books or guides that can help you out.

- **YouTube Tutorials:** YouTube is like a treasure trove of knowledge. You can find videos on just about anything! Whether it's learning to cook a new recipe, fixing a leaky faucet, or even mastering a new dance move, there's a video for it. Just type what you're curious about in the search bar, and off you go!

- **Library:** Remember the good old library? It's still there, and it's a fantastic place to explore. You can find books, magazines, and even classes on a wide range of topics. Plus, it's a peaceful place to spend some time.

- **Online Courses:** The internet is your friend, and there are many websites where you can take online courses. Websites like Coursera, Udemy, and Khan Academy offer courses on various subjects. You can learn at your own pace, and many of them are free!

- **Join a Club or Group:** If you want to learn something new and make friends at the same time, consider joining a local club or group. Whether it's a gardening club, a book club, or a knitting group, you'll have fun while learning.

- **Podcasts:** If you like listening, podcasts are a fantastic way to learn. There are podcasts on almost every topic you can think of. You can listen to them while you're cooking, walking, or just relaxing.

- **Volunteer:** Volunteering can be a great way to learn and give back to the community. You can volunteer at a local museum, animal shelter, or community center. You'll gain new skills and make a positive impact.

- **Online Forums:** If you have questions or want to discuss a topic, there are online forums and communities where you can join the conversation. Just Google your interest along with "forum" or "community," and you'll find a place to connect with others.

Remember, learning doesn't have to be a daunting task. It can be fun and exciting, and there are so many resources out there to help you along the way. So, go ahead, explore, practice, and enjoy the journey!

Unique Selling Points

★ **Daily Routine Approach:** "Balanced Living" takes a refreshingly different approach by presenting balance exercises as daily routines. Instead of feeling like a daunting task, readers can integrate these routines seamlessly into their lives. This user-friendly approach recognizes that consistency is key, and by framing exercises as routines, it encourages seniors to make balance a natural part of their daily routine.

★ **Mindfulness Integration:** What sets "Balanced Living" apart is its holistic approach. In addition to physical balance exercises, the book incorporates mindfulness practices. This combination transforms it into a comprehensive guide to overall well-being. It not only helps seniors improve their physical stability but also nurtures their mental and emotional health. By blending balance and mindfulness, the book acknowledges the interconnectedness of mind and body.

★ **"Balanced Living" strives for utmost clarity and accessibility.** To achieve this, each exercise is accompanied by soothing illustrations. These visual aids guide seniors through the routines with ease, making the book suitable for readers of all levels. The presence of clear, step-by-step illustrations ensures that seniors can confidently follow along and perform the exercises correctly.

★ **Holistic Well-being** Beyond the physical aspect of balance, "Balanced Living" recognizes that seniors have holistic needs. It goes beyond merely addressing physical balance and also focuses on mental and emotional equilibrium. The book offers guidance and practices to help seniors nurture their mental well-being, reduce stress, and enhance emotional resilience. This holistic approach acknowledges that true well-being encompasses various aspects of life.

In summary, "Balanced Living" is not just another exercise book for seniors. It stands out with its daily routine approach, mindfulness integration and commitment to holistic well-being. By offering a comprehensive and accessible guide, it empowers seniors to take charge of their balance, health, and overall quality of life.

Conclusion

Living: 5-Minute Daily Routines for Seniors" is an innovative and highly beneficial resource for seniors who are seeking to improve their balance, reduce stress, and enhance their overall quality of life. This book offers a practical and sustainable approach to well-being by blending daily routines, mindfulness practices, and soothing illustrations. With this holistic guide, seniors can achieve physical, mental, and emotional balance, paving the way for a more fulfilling and active aging experience.

The soothing illustrations throughout the book add a touch of artistry and make it a joy to read. They can also serve as visual aids for the mindfulness exercises, making the book both informative and visually pleasing. The ultimate goal is to help seniors maintain an active and vibrant lifestyle. By incorporating these daily routines, seniors can look forward to enjoying life to the fullest, staying engaged in their favorite activities, and pursuing new interests.

This nifty book is all about keeping it simple and making life sweeter. No fancy jargon or complicated stuff here. It's all about easy-peasy, practical ways to feel your best every day. We all know how important it is to stick to a routine. "Balanced Living" gives you super simple daily routines that take just five minutes. Yup, you read that right—five minutes! You can totally handle that. These routines are designed to help improve your balance, so you'll feel steady on your feet.

Stress got you down? Not anymore! This book introduces you to the world of mindfulness. It's like a mental spa day, and you can do it in just a few minutes. These practices will help you chill out, find your Zen, and wave goodbye to stress. Who doesn't love pretty pictures? "Balanced Living" is loaded with calming illustrations that make everything easier to understand. They'll put a smile on your face and help you stay relaxed.

Now, here's the best part: this book isn't just about your physical balance. It's about keeping your mind and heart in balance too. You know, the whole package! When you're balanced on the inside and outside, life gets a whole lot better.

So, whether you're a seasoned senior or just getting started on this aging adventure, "Balanced Living" is your ticket to a more awesome life. Give it a try, and you'll see that balance isn't just for acrobats; it's for all of us who want to enjoy life to the fullest.

Get ready to step into a world of simple daily routines, mindfulness, and beautiful illustrations that will help you feel better than ever. Don't wait; start living your best-balanced life today!